Few people realize that twe[...] discovery of the Dead Sea Scr[...], [...] of the same Essene teachings had already been uncovered. It began innocuously enough when an eighteen year old Valedictorian named Edmund Bordeaux Szekely gave a talk at his high school graduation ceremony entitled "Let St. Francis Sing In Your Heart." It so moved the Headmaster of the monastery, that he sent it to an old friend, Monsignor Mercati, the Prefect of the Vatican Archives in Rome, who after reading the paper, subsequently invited the young man to come study in the Vatican Archives.

The day they met, Mercati asked young Szekely why he wanted to study in the archives and Szekely told him of his "desire to know the source of St. Francis' knowledge." He later recalled the Monsignor's response was both "cryptic and fascinating…he told me that St. Francis was the ocean, and I must find the River nourishing it just as he did, and then I must look for the Stream. And then if I am firmly on the path, I will find the Source."

Szekely spent many months buried in ancient manuscripts and was even allowed access to off-limit areas within the 25 miles of book-shelves that lay beneath the Vatican. The Prefect even made special arrangements so Szekely could have full access to the Scriptorium at the Benedictine Monastery in Monte Cassino. There he poured over documentation about the life and teachings of Jesus that had never been seen; unexpurgated editions of the great historians Flavius Josephus, Philo and Plinius along with numerous other Latin classics. As Szekely put it:

"Many of these priceless works had generally been considered long lost, and I read and read through a treasure trove of unbelievable richness." He continues:

"I had found the source: Hebrew fragments of the Essene Gospel, the Aramaic version of which I had just read from the shelves of Monsignor Mercati's locked room."

Upon returning to the Vatican Mercati only had to see his face and he knew,

"You have found the source."

"How do you know?" young Szekely replied.

"Because, my son, you have that look."

At that point the young man could no longer hold back the tears.

"What shall I do father?" he cried.

The answer Monsignor Mercati gave him could very well change the world.

"Let St. Francis sing in your heart." the monsignor advised.

This book was inspired into being after Gene Wall Cole was introduced to the amazing life and the 80 plus books written by the late Edmund Bordeaux Szekely. Here's what one British writer Dion Byngham said in an article in the monthly journal "Health and Life," in July 1936, when referring to one of Mr. Szekely's books. He could just as easily have written the same review for Jesus' DieT...

"If the contents of a book could save our contemporary world, which is eddying and crashing to ruin, that book I believe has been written. If the contents of a book could redeem us as individuals from a common destiny of disease and death, that same book has appeared. If between the covers of a book might be found the sure path to creative peace, to superb health and beauty, to an optimal abundance of joy in life, let us open and read it. For if, while reading, we should perchance decide to live what we read, all these seeming miracles might assuredly happen."

Jesus' DieT
for
All the World

Gene Wall Cole

iv

ISBN 0-966-46448-6
Printed in the United States of America

A.I. Publishing
P.O. Box 344
Henrietta, N.C. 28076
e-mail awakening1@bellsouth.net
Website www.genewallcole.com
Office 828-657-5416

Contact information for Keynotes, Seminars, Workshops and Concerts with Gene Wall Cole turn to back page.

Table of Contents

Acknowledgments

I express special thanks:

To the thousands of readers of my multi-media first of its kind book, *The Chameleon*. Many of who have taken the time to write and share how reading it and listening to the accompanying music touched your lives. Also to the thousands of people who have attended my public seminars and concerts and have supported my Awakening Imaginations Foundation over the years. I feel this book is my way of saying thank you. Your support wasn't in vain.

To my surprise editor Pauline Kart, your ninety years of wisdom have been a true inspiration and you are a living example of what is possible.

To Ron (Kofi) Walker for your continued support and inspired graphics – you never cease to amaze me.

To Ann Walters for support in every manner conceivable while holding down the fort at Awakening Imaginations and allowing me the opportunity to help make the world a better place. I couldn't have done this without you!

To the hundreds of authors that have laid the groundwork for me on these important topics. I'll do my best to mention you all in the footnotes.

A special thanks to the late Edmund Bordeaux Szekely who led one of the most amazing and inspiring lives I could ever imagine. One of my goals in life is to make sure more of the world discovers you.

A special note of gratitude to the hundreds of reverends, and ministers who have entrusted me with their pulpits, and shared

viii

with me the wisdom, experience, strength and hope that comes from devoting ones' life to the spiritual path. To me you are some of the unsung heroes making a difference, one life at a time.

To all the volunteers and friends that have helped "Awakening Imaginations" take its message to the world. A very special thanks to Bill Campbell...thank you for your friendship as well as the added incentive! And most of all to my parents, Ben Nooe Cole and Jeanne Claire Wall, for conspiring to bring me into this world.

To my friend and collaborator Dr. Gail Bowdish for her decades of service as an emergency room doctor as well as her unwavering commitment to truth, even when it entails speaking truth to power.

Lastly, to those yet to be inspired by the vision behind Jesus' DieT... May these pages open your eyes and rock your world.

An extra special thanks to the team that helped give me a second wind on this marathon writing experience: Molly Wanning at Wanning Design for her classy design work; Sue Moran at Sue Moran Typography and Design for the detail that does make the difference; Patricia "Patticakes" from Hewlett Packard for reminding me as I remind others, that the good can often be the enemy of the great; Diane Baldwin for final editing and going beyond the call of duty; and Vivian Burgard from Moore Wallace for overseeing the final laps and putting it altogether for the world to see.

The Doctor's Prescription

Before we get into the meat of this diet (pun intended) let's consider an entirely new approach to how we look at food. The way our foods are currently categorized is part of the problem and we desperately need a solution. Obesity in the United States is now at epidemic proportions and the number of people suffering diabetes, cancer, heart attacks, strokes, as well as dozens of other preventable diseases is already off the chart. The old way of looking at food obviously isn't working. Unfortunately, the four basic food categories listed on packaging labels (protein, carbohydrates, fats and starches) merely denote the chemical composition of foods rather than a much more user-friendly differentiation such as life generating, life sustaining, life debilitating, or life destroying. This categorization is a more practical way of defining the effect of food on our bodies. To put it bluntly, the typical American diet promoted by 'The Great American Food Machine' consists primarily of either life-debilitating or life-destroying foods which literally slow down all of our body's processes while at the same time accelerating the processes of aging, disease and obesity. Period

As a student of medicine at Mayo Clinic, I was trained to think of the body as a machine, in the Newtonian physics model. In the ensuing years while seeing thousands of people as an emergency room physician, I have now come to understand the body from the perspective of quantum physics, which tells us that everything in the universe is energy, including our bodies. Food is energy, and vibrates at a certain frequency, and live foods vibrate at the highest frequencies which help promote healing. To the contrary, the processing of food lowers or destroys its vibrational frequencies, and subsequently that of our bodies, which then leads to disease. By following the suggestions in Jesus' DieT, you can promote self-healing by giving your body the life generating and life sustaining foods it needs not only to survive but to thrive.

I do believe that in God's Universe all things happen for a reason and every idea has its time and place. The time for Jesus' DieT is here and now. This book is based on a treasure trove of information that was first given 2000 years ago and rediscovered 75 years ago. It matters not what religious affiliation you may or may not have as this diet and the health benefits herein were meant to benefit every person on the planet. To your health!

Dr. Gail E. Bowdish, MD, FACEP
Fleet Surgeon, Great Lakes Cruising Club

Prologue

"Age doesn't always come with wisdom—it sometimes comes alone!" Author Unknown

This little book in your hands contains an accumulation of wisdom gathered from numerous sources; ancient wisdom as well as modern wisdom that can be used in three different ways to enrich your life. For many of you, it will be enough to consider it as **a simple diet book** on how to rapidly and safely lose all those extra pounds while teaching you a program for living prescribed by one of the world's greatest healers some 2000 years ago. Others of you, who view the body as the temple for the spirit, will see it as **a wake up call;** a book of revelation to attain maximum health and peace of mind that will guide you to that next step in your spiritual quest. And lastly, for the more curious and adventurous of you out there, this book will serve as **a roadmap** to help you solve for yourself one of the greatest 'whodunits' in history; a fascinating true story with all the ingredients of a great mystery.

It might seem odd to combine a diet book, a spiritual quest and a mystery all in one, but it is that very combination that has motivated thousands of people to dramatically change not only their bodies, but in many instances their entire lives for the better. Let me explain

I've been passionate about all three subjects most of my life, but it was only after I combined them that I found the inspiration to recreate myself. First, I've often found myself wanting to lose weight. I have tried various diet plans for the past 30 years from Weight Watchers, The Zone, Jenny Craig, South Beach Diet, and The Atkins Diet – especially diets that profess to give me more energy and mental clarity.

Second, my spiritual quest was inspired at age 18 by my first mentor, and has been an ongoing process ever since. My particular fascination has been with the path Jesus walked, as I was unable to resist the promise of his words "the things I do ye shall do and even greater things than these…." That search eventually led me to start a non-profit foundation where I've been using my gifts of music and humor to open hearts and plant seeds of wisdom, such as what you will find here. Over the past few years, I have found the best part of the job has been getting to meet and often break bread with others who have devoted their lives to "being about their father's business." That is where the first seeds of this book began to sprout.

Now there are many men and women who practice a spiritual and contemplative life, with their chief employment being to celebrate God and teach others how they may do so as well. This is highly commendable, but over the years I began to think how much more agreeable they would become in the eyes of man and God alike, if they would embrace a more balanced way of living; one that was an ornament of health and vitality. What a great example that would set for people to see their spiritual leaders enjoying constant health and happiness and attaining a great age. All this while becoming profoundly wise and useful in passing along their experience, strength and hope onto the upcoming generations. Instead, I have found they are mostly infirm, irritable and believe their ailments are trials sent to them by God.

I think they are mistaken.

I do not believe God wants humankind to be overweight, infirm, diseased and keeling over after only six and seven decades on this earth. Once I researched how many people have lived to be centurions and how they did it, I became thoroughly convinced that's not at all what was meant when we were admonished to "have life and have it more abundantly." *I believe that God would have us enjoy long life, health and happiness, but it's man himself, either through his ignorance or willful over-indulgence, that brings these ailments upon himself.* If those who profess to be our teachers on spiritual matters would set the example and treat the body as the temple it is intended to be, they would do much to pave the spiritual path for others to follow.

Third, I've had an insatiable quest for knowledge and adventure and been seeking out the questions to life since a young age. Family legend has it I got intoxicated for the first time at age four, though I can assure you that since I got such an early start, I used up my share in a hurry and have done these last two decades of research sober as a judge. It was my quest to solve some of the mystery around the life of Jesus that finally brought all three pieces together, and from which arose this book. The brilliance of this diet has been hidden from view for 1,930 years and I suspect the satisfaction you will get in shining some light on the mysterious 20 years of Jesus' life that are unaccounted for, will only be surpassed by what you will soon get from looking in the mirror.

Introduction

"I care not much for a man's religion whose dog or cat are not the better for it."

– Abraham Lincoln

Let me start by answering a few of the more obvious questions such as what inspired me to write this book, and why should you be interested in what my research has uncovered? Also, who am I, and where did I discover all the amazing details I'm about to share? And lastly, if it's all true, why haven't you heard about it before now? The short answer is, I wrote it because two of our founding fathers and former U.S. presidents inspired me. Let me explain. Few people realize the enormous freedom that opens up with the three simple words "I don't know." It's probably because that acceptance allows the space for a true knowingness to then appear within the humility. That's why some people are so much better grandparents than they were parents. The fact is, all anyone really *knows* for sure is that an extraordinary man named Jesus walked the earth some 2000 years ago. Exactly what he said and what he did and how he meant for it to be used in our daily lives, no one can know for certain since none of us were there. In the past two centuries alone, so many glaring discrepancies have been pointed out about what is known as the Biblical 'canon,' that many of our founding fathers, even former Presidents such as Abraham Lincoln and Thomas Jefferson felt compelled to speak on the subject.

Not only did they warn of the great peril that *'belief without reason'* could lead to, but in Jefferson's case he actually offered some alternative perspective. His body of work on the subject

eventually became known as "The Jefferson Bible"[1] and until
recently, was handed out to all new members of Congress as the
Congressional Bible they received when first taking office. I
sincerely doubt that more than a handful of our representatives in
Washington have ever taken the time to read it though, as
politicians back then weren't so much interested in being politically
correct as in telling the whole truth and nothing but the truth. I
daresay Lincoln and Jefferson would both be shocked to see how
those teachings have been used for political purposes. Here's a
sampling from each of them that first motivated me to dig deeper.
First Mr. Jefferson:

"Among the sayings and discourses imputed to him (Jesus) by his
biographers, I find many passages of fine imagination, correct
morality, and of the most lovely benevolence; and others again of
so much ignorance, so much absurdity, so much untruth,
charlatanism, and imposture, that such contradictions should have
proceeded from the same being."

Ignorance, absurdity, charlatanism – some pretty strong words
from one of our most learned and respected founding fathers.

While it's true that the theological inconsistencies of Christianity
have become a cross to bear, I have recently found something high
above all the theology that has brought back the teachings of Jesus
in a way I could have never imagined before. I'm speaking of the
teachings of Jesus found at the Dead Sea in 1945, and those found
even earlier in the secret vaults of the Vatican by Edmund Bordeaux
Szekely in the mid 1920's. That is what this book is based upon
and where this diet originates; the mouth of Jesus himself. I believe
Jefferson referred to them as "passages of fine imagination, correct
morality and the most lovely benevolence." Within the words of
Jesus that were uncovered lie not only an amazingly effective diet,
but also a beautiful ethical system by which to live our lives as well.
Within the spirit of Christianity there is a moral code and way of
living that has eternal vigor and vitality, if people could only hear
the words of Jesus himself that have been hidden away within the

---

[1] Jefferson, Thomas "The Jefferson Bible —The Life and Morals of Jesus of Nazareth"
1904, Beacon Press

Vatican vaults: Words such as:
> "I tell you truly, that the scripture is the work of man, but life and all its hosts are the work of God… all living things are nearer to God than the scriptures which are without life."[2]

On January 24th, 1813 Jefferson wrote in a letter to another one of our Presidents John Adams.

> "The whole history of these books (the gospels) is so defective and doubtful that it seems vain to attempt minute inquiry into it; and such tricks have been played with their text, and with the text of other books relating to them, that we have a right, from that cause, to entertain much doubt what parts of them are genuine. In the New Testament there is internal evidence that parts of it proceeded from an extraordinary man; and that other parts are of the fabric of very inferior minds. It is as easy to separate those parts, as to pick out diamonds from dunghills."

It was Jefferson's admonition to pick out "diamonds from dunghills" that particularly motivated my research. Truth be known, I literally found myself in tears when I first discovered these writings and experienced for myself the authenticity and power behind the words. I have no doubt that many of you will have the same reaction, as well as the same dramatic results once you start to put them into practice. Here are the thoughts of yet another President on looking at the modern day 'canon' as being inerrant:

> *"My earlier views of the unsoundness of the Christian scheme of salvation and the human origin of the scriptures have become clearer and stronger with advancing years and I see no reasons for thinking I shall ever change them."*
> *– Abraham Lincoln (letter to Judge J. Wakefield)*

Having said that, it is almost impossible for any thinking man to not realize *something* spectacular happened 2000 years ago. Unfortunately it's something the rest of the world has been arguing about ever since. Everyone has an opinion and their preferred beliefs on the subject, but the reality is, no *one really knows what happened.* Not Billy Graham, not Oral Roberts, not King James, not even Mel Gibson – there's no one that really knows for sure,

---

[2] Edmund Bordeaux Szekely "The Essene Origins of Christianity" IBS

and if they claim they do, you'd be wise to start backing towards the door.

What we *can* know for certain, is that some beliefs need to change as more knowledge is *un*covered and facts *dis*covered, while other beliefs need to be discarded altogether in the light of new information. Everyone once *believed* the world was flat, but we now *know* otherwise and have discarded that belief. People once *believed* the earth was the center of the universe, until the startling discovery by Galileo that the sun didn't rotate around the earth, so we now *know* it's the other way around. Consider what an outrageous and frightening claim that had to be to the ecclesiastical powers of the time. Remember they depended on the unquestioned assumptions that had been held for the previous 1600 years to hold sway over their *believers*. By the way, the church's response to Galileo at the time was to pronounce him a heretic for expressing those beliefs and condemn him to death for his discovery. (For those not quite up to date, in 1991 the Vatican finally admitted Galileo had been right all along – "*Only 400 some-odd years late but hey, better late than never,*" remarked one of the Episcopal churches most learned Bishops.) The fact remains, Galileo *knew* something to be true though he nearly lost his life for expressing it. *Knowing* the truth once again wins out over merely *believing* you know the truth.

People once *believed* that lightning had to do with a God named Thor who hung out on Mount Olympus, but we now *know* otherwise. How about Sir Isaac Newton (1643-1727) who recognized that we live in an orderly world and totally debunked the superstitions of the majority of people who *believed* in the invasive power of a supernatural God who would punish us with earthquakes and floods. More and more people now *know* the world works on fixed laws, so the *belief* that weather, sickness and wars are divine interventions had to be questioned and eventually discarded.

The *belief* in theories like relativity, gravity, and the speed of light only became accepted as known facts over time. Many of us might not understand the details, but there are enough others that *know* them to be true that we can trust what they say. I could go on and on with the discoveries of Darwin, Einstein, and Stephen Hawkings that we now *know* to be true which further alienate worn out *beliefs*, but the point is, when it comes to beliefs, as Jefferson emphatically warned us, we need to be careful.

The only thing we can know for certain about the Bible is that it is more like a painting and not a photograph of Jesus and the times in which he lived. Regardless of how uncomfortable it might be to admit it, there is no religion superior to the truth. Elaine Pagels in "Beyond Belief" described this longing for the truth as "the impulse to seek God" that "overflows the narrow banks of a single tradition."[3]

Jesus himself warned his disciples:

> "Seek not the law in your scriptures for the law is life. Whereas the scripture is dead... I tell you truly, that the scripture is the work of man, but life and all its hosts are the work of our God."[4]

Now to the question of who is this author that you should take 'shekels' out of your pocket and time out of your life to read this little book of wisdom. For starters, I'm just an average Joe who happens to have an insatiable curiosity for knowledge. Knowledge of any stripe! God gave me a good brain and I love to exercise it. An average Joe who has always rooted for the little guy; the underdog, and believed in the idea of fair play. A "let's have a fair fight and may the best man win" kind of Joe! The kind of Joe who gets bugged because our national pastime has evolved into something the New York Yankees can buy most of the time, and wants to know what can be done to fix it. A Joe who's curious about the mysteries on this planet we call home as well as the human condition. A Joe who wants all the knowledge available on how to live right and eat right to maximize the full potential of being human by taking proper care of this temple I have been blessed with. There's little that doesn't pique my curiosity as I just love to learn. I'm the kind of Joe who wants to go everywhere, do everything and experience all life has to offer. My search for knowledge is insatiable, *especially regarding wisdom others might*

---

[3] Ibid, note no. 6
[4] Edmund Bordeaux Szekely "Essene Gospel of Peace"

want to keep hidden from an Average Joe. That's my real passion.

My prayer is that every person reading this will hold off any preconceived notions and not only listen but hear what was discovered in 1925 and 1947 before they make up their minds and dismiss these findings out of hand. If you can keep an open mind and use the wisdom garnered here, the least you'll do is lose all those unwanted pounds and gain back your health and vitality – that's a guarantee!

Again, for those of you who either want a short-cut or don't have that insatiable curiosity to know the source of all this information before starting to use it, you might want to jump ahead to the chapter entitled *'How It Works.'* For the rest of you, delve into solving some of the 'whodunit' without further ado.

The Roadmap
The Journey Begins

I've always found it a bit incredulous that with all the detailed history written during the time of Jesus, 20 years of his life could remain almost a total mystery. What did he do during this time, where did he go, who were his teachers, who were his friends? I'd heard rumors all my life that Jesus had studied with the Essenes (arguably the most unique brotherhood in the history of mankind) during those accounted years, but no one ever seemed to have specifics on either the rumor or about the Essenes themselves. I found this especially disconcerting when there was so much information available about the other two major Jewish sects of the time, the Sadducees and the Pharisees. When you start to consider that the Essenes were much older and certainly the most respected of all the Jewish sects back then, it becomes even more of a mystery worth unraveling.

Much of what I've discovered has been available to those willing to seek it out for 75 years, but when it was first released there was only the word of Edmund Bordeaux Szekely, the man who first uncovered it as to its authenticity. Combine that, with the worldwide interest and radio coverage of the Scopes trial in 1925 (considered by many to be the trial of the century), the ensuing uproar about Darwin's theory of evolution, and it's not surprising that Szekely's findings would be given faint attention. In retrospect, many people saw this as 'the beginning of the end' for the tattered and frayed belief in the Bible as the *inerrant* word of God. For those not familiar with the Scopes trial, here is an exchange between Clarence Darrow, arguably the greatest defense attorney

ever, and three time presidential candidate William Jennings
Bryant.

Q: "You have given considerable study to the Bible, haven't you,
   Mr. Bryant?"
A: "Yes, sir; I have tried to ... But, of course, I have studied it
   more as I have become older than when I was a boy."
Q: "Do you claim then that everything in the Bible should be
   literally interpreted?"
A: "I believe everything in the Bible should be accepted as it is
   given there ..."

Darrow continued to question Bryan on the actuality of Jonah
and the whale, Joshua's making the sun stand still and the Tower of
Babel, as Bryant began to have more difficulty answering.

Q: "Do you think the earth was made in six days?"
A: "Not six days of 24 hours ... My impression is they were
   periods ..."
Q: "Now, if you call those periods, they may have been a very
   long time?"
A: "They might have been."
Q: "The creation might have been going on for a very long
   time?"
A: "It might have continued for millions of years ..."

Which is exactly what Darwin had been saying all along.
It wasn't until two decades later (in 1945) that we would
discover The Gospel of Thomas along with more than 50 other
early Christian texts unknown since antiquity. In them we would
find many of the same accounts of Jesus and the Essenes that
Szekely had found in the Vatican vaults in the mid 1920's. With
the discovery of the Dead Sea Scrolls in corroboration with
Szekely's findings 20 years earlier, we can no longer ignore the
evidence as it has become overwhelming as to its authenticity.
It's no exaggeration to think that the discoveries Szekely made,
combined with the writings found in the Dead Sea Scrolls, could
very well change the course of human history. Unfortunately, few
people are aware of their existence or their potential significance.

Jesus' DieT... is my intention to remedy that. Once I put the two
discoveries together I was flabbergasted. The obvious authenticity,
the depth, the clarity and the potential meaning of these discoveries
felt like one of the greatest treasures on earth. In light of what has
happened in our world recently, my first thoughts were "I wish a
lot more people were aware of these findings." Unfortunately, just
as the Scopes trial had to drown out Szekely's findings in the mid
20's, I suspect the end of World War II was so monumental, so
huge, that anything else of importance that happened during that
time, had little chance of getting the attention it deserved. When
you consider the world had just experienced more fear and
witnessed more death and destruction than anytime in human
history, it's not hard to understand. Combine the enormous
anguish of millions of people dying, with the experience of
overwhelming joy at the defeat of Hitler, and there would have
been little air left for anything else. (Certainly not new information
on a moral code and a way of living found in a gold-mine that had
been caving in for centuries from the weight of its own dogma and
prejudice.) Unfortunately, discoveries about the Essenes such as
those found by Szekely and in the Dead Sea Scrolls would have
been relegated to the back pages after its initial exposure.

At one point in my research, I went to the main library in Ann
Arbor, Michigan (home to one of the nation's leading universities),
and only after getting an interlibrary loan could I find two of the
Szekely books. Both were several states away and had to be
borrowed through the interlibrary system. I was told at the time
there were only 100 copies of the book in the entire country. Then
as I learned of more titles by Szekely (80 books in all) I tried again,
and this time I found out the new book I requested only had 7
copies in the American library system and was told it would be
almost impossible to get.

What was going on? This was starting to remind me of the 1000
year period in history when it was considered a crime punishable
by death to even have a copy of the "Bible" in your possession. I
already knew much of the history of how the Church fathers had
constructed the early 'canon' to stabilize the emerging Christian
church, and in the process had suppressed many of its spiritual

resources. Now I had some of those same resources in my hands. I
then began to envision what the world would be like if these other
books hadn't been suppressed.

The Plot Thickens

These teachings have come to us independently from numerous
sources. Some were found in the Vatican vaults; some in an earthen
jar found near The Dead Sea where they had lain undisturbed for
1600 years; some are from historians that were contemporaries of
Jesus; and some from the authenticated Gospel of Thomas. Within
the authenticated manuscripts already found, there are dialogues,
sayings, and rituals written during the 1ˢᵗ century that are attributed
to Jesus and his disciples. Specifically, Jesus told his disciples in
private about not only feeding one's soul but also one's body,
which he constantly refers to as 'the temple.' Some of it was written
by the apostle of Jesus we now know as "Doubting Thomas" (the
nickname given him in the Gospel of John). Since the writings of
Thomas and The Essene Gospel of Peace are two of the texts that
have been suppressed by the church, this seems like a good place to
begin unraveling our mystery. In setting the table for the metaphoric feast you're about to enjoy, I will first offer a few clues to
that 'whodunit' so you'll know these are the actual teachings or
(diet plan if you prefer) of Jesus. If you're an atheist or an agnostic
or simply bought this book to lose weight and get healthy, don't
worry, even if you don't believe where these teachings originated,
they still work and you'll still get the desired physical results in the
very least. Like Jesus said "By their works ye shall know them."

Let's begin with the discovery of The Gospel of Thomas as it has
numerous similarities with the Gospel of John. This extraordinary
piece of the puzzle becomes all the more important when you
realize the underpinning for the entire Christian movement since
the mid-third century are based on the writings found in the
Gospel of John. In fact, most Biblical scholars agree *John is the lens
from which most people view the three synoptic gospels of Matthew,
Mark and Luke.* (For God so loved the world…[1]) Once you read

---

[1] Holy Bible, John 3:16

the writings of Thomas, it becomes apparent that the author(s) of
The Gospel of John wrote it some time afterwards as a direct
counter to the interpretation Thomas gives Jesus' message. In other
words, a strong case can be made that much of what is written in
the gospel of John is actually a polemic against the teachings of
Thomas.

"Written in the heat of controversy to defend certain views and
oppose others"[2] is how Princeton professor Elaine Pagels describes
her understanding of The Gospel of John after studying the Book
of Thomas.

It seems likely the two men and their respective camps were very
much rivals at the end of the first century as whoever wrote the
Gospel of John describes Thomas quite negatively as one who had
no faith, doubted everything, and who understood little. The more
time one spends reading the two gospels side by side, the more it
seems likely there was enmity if not downright jealousy between
the author(s) of The Gospels of John and Thomas. Especially when
you note that the Gospels of both Luke and Mathew, which were
written many years earlier than John, also refer to the apostle
Thomas, but simply have him as another one of the disciples noting
nothing in particular. Now for the first time we have him as a full-
bodied character.

It's likely that each of the disciple's respective camps believed
their man was the favorite of Jesus as did numerous sects splintered
off from the original teachings. All claimed to be inspired by the
Holy Spirit. Prophecy, speaking in tongues, revelations, visions, and
the power to heal, were all contentious subjects with some like
Gaius in Rome who argued that all genuine revelations ended with
the close of the apostolic age. Other groups disagreed vehemently.
It becomes obvious the amount of discord between the dozens of
various camps was quite intense, and that's putting it mildly.

Both Gospels of John and Thomas begin with the secret teachings
Jesus gave his disciples, using the same unique language to tell the
same stories. But it's their interpretations that are quite different. In
the Book of Thomas the text calls them "secret sayings which the

---

[2] Elaine Pagels, "Beyond Belief", 2003, Random House

living Jesus spoke" to his disciples, not the public teaching that he
gave to the world. It's even written on the ancient script itself:
"Didymus Judas Thomas wrote them down."[3] *This statement alone
is startling* as no other Gospel writings have ever stated who
actually wrote them, and numerous biblical scholars are convinced
that none of the writers of the existing four gospels ever actually
met Jesus. If that's the case, *these could very well be as close to the
source as we've ever seen!*

"Secret teachings" Thomas calls them because they are for his
disciples who have gone to a "different level." Similarly, when John
tells what happened after Judas' betrayal, he inserts five chapters of
unique intimate dialogue between Jesus and the disciples. In one
section of John the disciples keep asking questions like "tell us what
to do – what diet shall we observe? Should we give to charity?
How should we pray?" Jesus answers them very differently in
Thomas:

"Do not tell lies and do not do what you hate. For all things are
plain in the sight of heaven."

Just like what we find in John, this is where Jesus asks the
disciples "Who am I?" To paraphrase, Peter answers "like a
righteous messenger." Matthew answers "Like a wise philosopher
(rabbi)." But when Thomas answers "Master, my mouth is wholly
incapable of saying whom you are like."

Jesus replies:

"I am not your master, because you have drunk, and have
become drunk from the same stream I measured out."

Jesus then takes Thomas aside and reveals three sayings so secret
they cannot be written down, not even later in his Book of
Thomas. Then when Thomas returns to his companions they
asked, "what did he say to you?" Thomas replies:

"If I tell you even one of the things he told me, you will pick up
stones and throw them at me and a fire will come out of the stones
and burn you up."[4]

Thomas describes Jesus' message is that *every person has the light
of God within and that Jesus is a manifestation of the divine light*

---

[3] Gospel of Thomas 1 in NHI 118; Elaine Pagels "Beyond Belief", 2003 Random House
[4] Gospel of Thomas 50 NHI 125

that came into being at the beginning of time. He goes on to say
*'The Good News' (the gospel) is that so are you and that everyone
comes from that same divine light.*

"Yes, I am the son of God" Jesus says, "but you too are also the
child of God when you come to recognize who you
really are."

Thomas interprets that the 'Kingdom of God' (which is the topic
of Jesus' teachings according to Mathew and Luke) is that the
divine light is within everything, not just human beings.

"The kingdom is inside you and outside you" says Jesus. "Split a
piece of wood and I am there. Lift up the rock and you will find
me there."

According to **both** John and Thomas "the kingdom of heaven is
already here" as a continuing spiritual reality. In The Book of
Thomas Jesus says "whoever finds the interpretation of these words
will not taste death." But he warns the disciples that the search will
both 'disturb and astonish' you.

"If you bring forth what is within you, what you bring forth will
save you. If you do not bring forth what is within you, what you do
not bring forth will destroy you."

There are many other reasons to discern that after Jesus died,
a rivalry and even jealousy came between these two disciples and
their respective camps. Most biblical scholars have been puzzled
that there are a number of stories in the Gospel of John that
stand alone or actually contradict the other three Gospels of
Matthew, Mark and Luke, such as John referring to Jesus'
disrupting the money changers as his (first) public act, whereas
Matthew, Mark and Luke all say that this was his (last) public
act which then led to his arrest and the high priests seeking to
kill him. John explains the arrest as being caused by Jesus'
raising of Lazarus from the dead, which no other Gospel writer
ever makes reference to, despite the fact that was one of the
most dramatic miracles Jesus performed.

Another obvious discrepancy concerning the disciple Thomas is
that both Luke[5] and Mathew[6] specify that after the crucifixion

[5] Luke 24:33-36
[6] Matthew 28:10

Jesus appeared to all 11 disciples except for Judas Escariot: "conferred on 'the eleven' the power of the Holy Spirit." In marked contrast John alone says: "Thomas called 'the twin'....was not with them when Jesus came."[7]

According to John's gospel, this meeting was crucial as this is when Jesus designated them apostles as he "breathed upon them" and later delegated them to forgive sins. The implication is clear that John wants us to believe Thomas isn't a true apostle since he had not received "the spirit." Then John goes on to his "coup de' grace" with the story of 'doubting Thomas,' which is all most people remember today; "Unless I see the nails... I will not believe" etc.[8] None of the other Gospels support this at all, only in John.

This is really where the mystery plot thickens. Who decided which of the many written teachings were to be canonized and which were to be burned? Who actually made the decisions that led to the compilation of what we now regard as The Holy Bible? Where did they get their authority and why did they choose one teaching over another?

It's a fascinating trail of clues, but I'll just give you the abbreviated version for now. For those readers particularly excited about learning all the details while solving the 'whodunit,' I would be remiss to not only start you out with Szekely's "Origin Of Christianity" and "The Essene Gospel of Peace," but with Elaine Pagels "Beyond Belief" as well. I have found hundreds of other authors that have done extensive research and found historical documents of all the various factions and councils and palace intrigues that occurred back then, but Pagels has definitely done her homework. Here's a bit of the history that motivated me to keep digging deeper and deeper.

At the end of the second century in Provincial Gaul, a Bishop of Lyon named Irenaeus became the first to promote John as the one true gospel among all the other teachings that were circulating at the time. As a young man he had witnessed much persecution in Lyons where he lived and had seen 'Christists' (the early name of the various factions of Jesus before the term 'Christian' replaced it)

---

[7] John 20:24
[8] John 20:19-23

assaulted, beaten, stoned and strangled, tortured in public and even torn apart by wild animals.[9] At one point a number of the 'Christist' prisoners wrote a letter to Marcus Aurelius, the emperor, and had asked Irenaeus to deliver it to Rome for them, which he did. Upon arriving, he found groups and factions on every side that challenged his understanding of the Gospel and many who even thought it was heresy. Irenaeus was even more distressed to learn from an old friend named Florinus, who like himself had studied with Polycarp, that an increasing number of educated Christians were moving in other directions from his own as well.[10] When Irenaeus returned home, he found many of his own group had been slaughtered in the public square and many in his own flock were now splintered into various groups, each claiming to be inspired by the Holy Spirit. Keep in mind there were many people in the first generation of readers (90-130 c.e.) that disagreed on whether The Gospel of John was a true Gospel at all,[11] but Irenaeus was convinced his belief was the correct one.

Irenaeus is responsible for forging a middle ground between all the factions, many who believed in revelation and many who didn't. "How can we tell the difference between the word of God and mere human words?" he asked.[12] Though Irenaeus never used the term 'canon' he was eventually able to consolidate his flock under what he called the "four formed gospel" in what is now part of France. It's interesting to note that not one of Irenaeus's three most revered mentors: Bishop Polycarp of Smyrna, the martyr Ignatius who was bishop of Antioch, nor Justin Martyr, the Christian philosopher in Rome whom Irenaeus particularly admired, seem to have known of John's Gospel at all, as none of them ever mentioned it.[13] One person who definitely didn't believe the true Gospel was in the teachings of John, was the Roman

[9] W.H.C. Friend, "Martyrdom and Persecution in the Early Church (Oxford, 1965: New York pgs.)

[10] Eusebius, "Historia Ecclesiate 5.20.4; Elaine Pagels, "Beyond Belief" , 2003 Random House

[11] Maurice F. Wiles "The Spiritual Gospel", Cambridge, 1960; C.H. Dodd "Interpretation of the 4th Gospel" Cambridge 1953

[12] Irenaneus, AH, 2.15.8: Elaine Pagels "Beyond Believe," 2003, Random House

[13] Koester, "Ancient Christian Gospel" ; See also J.N. Sanders "The Fourth Gospel in the Early Church" Cambridge 1943 and Maurice Wiles, "Spiritual Gospel," Elaine Pagels, "Beyond Belief"

teacher Gaius who not only called it heretical, but charged that it had actually been written by John's worst enemy the heretic Cerinthus.[14]

Nevertheless, Irenaeus's effort to consolidate obviously caught on as it led to one of the big events in the early Christian movement, actually helping put an end to much of the early Christian persecution. On Oct. 28, 312 a Bishop in Palestine named Eusebius of Caesarea gained the allegiance of the pagan emperor Constantine by converting him to Christianity.[15] Unfortunately, this practical military leader chose only to recognize the largest and most powerful of the numerous sects of that time, which was the same one that followed the tenets of John. A few years after he was converted, Emperor Constantine gathered a council together on the Turkish coast at a place called Nicaea, that officially named this particular group of writings "the legitimate and most Holy Catholic Church."[16] There was much heated debate in the council with some delegates even walking out in protest as there were literally dozens of rivaling factions by this time. This would later become known as the Nicene Creed and to this day still defines the faith for many Christians.

The political pressures the newly converted emperor brought to bear were amazing as he even offered tax relief and tax exemptions to clergy who qualified, while threatening to increase the taxes of anyone from the other "Christists" sects or those founding "heretical churches" as he called them.[17] Constantine also delegated Bishops from only his sect to the position of distributing the grain supply as well as other basic necessities which became another powerful incentive as you can imagine.

Now that the emperor had given his official stamp of approval, anyone who challenged the Nicene Creed was seen as challenging the orthodoxy of the emperor himself.[18] Besides losing out on tax relief and grain subsidies, opposing the emperor wasn't something

[14] Irenaneus, "Libros Quinque Adversus Haereses" 3.3.4, Cambridge, 1851
[15] Eusebius "Vita Constantinae" 1.26-29
[16] Eusebius "Historia Ecclesiae" 10.6
[17] Codex Theodosius 19.5.1
[18] Barnes "Constantine and Eusebius" 213 and Elaine Pagels "Beyond Belief," 2003, Random House

many were willing to publicly do. Remember they didn't live in a Democracy back then.

Though there are many well documented struggles leading up to his declaration, in the spring of 367, Athanasius, the Bishop of Alexandria, named the 27 books we now have in the New Testament as the only legitimate ones. At the same time he ordered all the other books, writings, gospels and supporting documents burned as he was determined to consolidate power under his leadership as the single most powerful Bishop in Egypt. This collection of books that we now call the 'canon' is what the Bishop of Alexandria thought would work for that purpose and he called them at the time, the "springs of salvation." All others books were to be destroyed as they were "apocryphal and taught blasphemy."

This is the earliest known list of the 27 books that would later make up our current Bible."[19] This is also when someone, probably monks from the monastery at St. Pachomius, took copies of the other teachings that had been banned (probably the manuscripts from their monastery library) and sealed them in a six foot jar and then buried them at Nag Hammadi. There they remained until an Egyptian villager named Muhammad Ali stumbled upon them some 1600 years later.

To further illustrate the reality of how our current Bible came to be and the importance of 'knowing rather than simply believing' something is true, let's jump ahead to 1611 when the King James Version was published. The reason I chose this version as an example is twofold. First, because it can make a legitimate claim to be the greatest work of prose in the English language with or without sales as the bellwether. And secondly, because a wonderful work by Adam Nicholson has recently been written describing the exact process the King James Version went through as well as the names of the fifty-four men who compiled it.[20]

Here's Nicholson describing the process to an interviewer on NPR: "I know there are a lot of people that would like to believe

[19] Athanasius, Festal Letter 39; Martin Tetz "Athanasius;" Brackke "Canon Formation and Social Conflict"
[20] Adan Nicholson, "God's Secretaries" How the King James Bible was Written, 2003, Harper Collins

that what we read in the King James Version of the Bible is a work
of inspiration by divinely inspired men…" "Not at all," he says "it
was extremely, tightly, totally organized" by a "modern
administrator," a bureaucratic Archbishop of Canterbury named
Richard Bancroft. Nicholson jokingly referred to it as being much
more like "the Manhattan Project" with a central institution type
government.

The rules for this bureaucracy were set up by Bancroft himself
and there is a copy of the original rules in Nicholson's book. He
reminds us there were 48 translators assigned into six committees,
two each in Oxford, Cambridge, and Westminster, with eight
people on each with a director. Each member translated his section
of the Bible, then showed it to the other eight members in his sub-
committee who had to approve it, before it was then sent on to the
central overseeing committee for approval. After the Central
Overseeing Committee approved each book, they were then sent to
Westminster and then finally on to the Archbishop and the King for
their approval. Changes of course were made all along the line.

There's little reason to believe it was much different 1300 years
earlier with Emperor Constantine and Bishop Irenaeus taking the place
of King James and the Archbishop of Cantebury – two political
administrators making the final decisions as to what would be deemed
as Holy Scripture. Well, actually there were a couple of other
differences. For one thing, Constantine and his cronies were a lot less
organized and a lot more politically motivated as their decisions would
actually be death warrants for many that didn't agree with them. Also,
they were choosing which books and teachings by which authors and
apostles out of the dozens if not hundreds of existing sects came closest
to supporting their narrow beliefs and political agendas. While on the
other hand, King James' group was simply deciding to either leave in,
take out, or change certain *words and phrases* as opposed to which
books and authors made the final cut. To be changing words and
phrases that are already of such questionable origin, hardly lends the
process any more credibility. To believe the King James version is the
inerrant and only word of God, seems to be a lot like "rearranging seats
on the Titanic," either way the ship is already full of holes and is going
down!

The Road Continues
Light At The End Of The Tunnel

Let's leap frog up to the early twentieth century before the tremendous Dead Sea discoveries in 1945. Few people realize that twenty-five years earlier, many of the same Essene teachings found in the Dead Sea Scrolls had already been uncovered. It began innocuously enough when an eighteen year old named Edmund Bordeaux Szekely gave a talk as Valedictorian at his high school graduation ceremonies. The talk he had prepared was entitled "Let St. Francis Sing In Your Heart." It seems that the talk so moved the Headmaster of the monastery, Monsignor Mondik, that he decided to send it to his old friend, Monsignor Mercati at the Vatican, who just happened to be the Prefect of the Vatican Archives. Mercati also loved the paper and subsequently invited young Szekely to come study in the Vatican Archives in Rome. There, Szekely met Monsignor Mercati for the first time. This fateful meeting would not only change his own life, but possibly the entire Christian world forever, as Mercati eventually allowed him access to a secret section of the 25 miles of bookshelves that was normally locked and off limits.

The day they first met, Monsignor Mercati asked him why he wanted to study in the archives and young Szekely told him of his "desire to know the source of St. Francis' knowledge." He later recalled Monsignor Mercati's response was both "cryptic and fascinating….he told me that: 'St. Francis was the Ocean, and I must find the River nourishing it, just as he did. Then I must look for the Stream. And then, if I am firmly on the Path I will find the Source.¹' "

---

[1] Edmond Bordeaux Szekely "Search For The Ageless, Vol. 1" International Biogenic Society

With the assistance of a French monk who translated both
Hebrew and Aramaic,[2] Szekely spent many months studying in the
Vatican vaults and then later at the Benedictine Monastery in
Monte Cassino where he found documentation about the life and
teachings of Jesus that had never been seen. Thanks to a letter
Monsignor Mercati wrote on his behalf, the Abbot at Monte
Cassino allowed him access to the vitrines there in the Scriptorium
where he was able to pore over unexpurgated editions of the great
historians Flavius Josephus, Philo and Plinius along with numerous
other Latin classics. As Szekely puts it:

> "Many of these priceless works had generally been considered
> long lost, and I read and read through a treasure trove of
> unbelievable richness." He continues:

> "I had found the source: Hebrew fragments of the Essene
> Gospel, the Aramaic version of which I had just read from the
> shelves of Monsignor Mercati's locked room. I knew now the
> origin of the inner light that shone from that beloved figure
> (Mercati), and I perceived in a flash of awareness, the heroic
> measure of his silence. Now, should I be silent, too?"[3] he asked
> himself.

Upon returning to the Vatican, Mercati only had to see his face
and he knew,

"You have found the source."

"How do you know?" young Szekely replied.

"Because, my son, you have that look."

At that point the young man could no longer hold back the tears.
"What shall I do father?" he cried.

The answer Monsignor Mercati gave him could very well change
the world.

"Let St. Francis sing in your heart." The monsignor advised.

"Jesus DieT.." was inspired in part, by Szekely's accounts of the
next several decades of doing just that, "letting St. Francis sing in
his heart." It has dramatically changed not only my world, but also
the million people that Szekely managed to touch through his
books and clinics over the next 75 years. Szekely's also known for
founding the first health spa in America called "The Golden Door"

[2] Edmond Bordeaux Szekely "Search For The Ageless, Vol. 1" International Biogenic Society
[3] Ibid

in California, and was teaching much of the diet I've written about half a century ago. Unfortunately, a million people is just a drop in the bucket with what those discoveries could and should be doing. In describing where Jesus' DieT... was uncovered, I hope I've given enough clues so that those readers wishing to delve further are inspired to proceed with great enthusiasm. But for those who simply want to learn a great way to lose weight while looking and feeling healthier than you probably have in years, without further ado please come sit with me at our metaphoric table, for our banquet is set and it's time to feast on the truth.

A Simple Diet Plan

"We must never permit the voice of humanity within us to be silenced. It is man's sympathy with all creatures that first makes him truly a man....Any religion which is not based on a respect for life is not a true religion...Until he extends his circle of compassion to all living things, man will not himself find peace."
Albert Schweitzer– Nobel Peace Prize winner

Because of the volatility in our world concerning all things "religious" and because these teachings are truly meant for everyone, I decided to keep the focus of this book on a part of the teachings that everyone, regardless of race, color, creed, nationality, religious orientation or political affiliation, could relate to, and that is:

<u>diet, noun</u>

1a. Habitual nourishment 1b. the kind and amount of food prescribed for a person or animal for a special reason
2. Something provided (especially habitually). A diet of Broadway shows
3. Regimen or game plan for attaining optimum health in all areas of life

<u>diet, verb</u>

1. to eat sparingly according to prescribed rules
2. Taking contrary actions concerning one's food intake
3. Re-examining the role food plays in one's life
4. The modern obsession of losing weight to look better which often leads to feeling better about oneself, and who knows

maybe even ending up with a new wardrobe or at least fitting
into the old one (Antonym – gorge, indulge, Yo-Yo)
diet, adjective
reduced in calories. a *diet* soft drink

I figured there aren't many people who couldn't relate to
something in there. With Jesus' DieT... we'll be taking a two-fold
approach and look at diet as both a noun (game plan/regimen), and
a verb (taking an action) to get our desired results. My observation
on diets over the years is that much of the industrialized world
seems to always be on one, and the other half looks like they could
use one. As I mentioned earlier, there are many good reasons
beyond just looking and feeling better to incorporate Jesus' DieT
into your life, but I'll resist the urge to go into them now and keep
this section simply about weight and health.

The medical community is now predicting that with the
enormous increase of obesity and lack of physical fitness in this
generation of children, that obesity will overtake smoking as the
number one most costly and damaging problem in America. Here's
a quote from Julie Gerberding, director of the Centers for Disease
Control and Prevention, "We just recalculated the actual causes of
death in the U.S. and we did see that obesity moved up very close
to tobacco, and is almost the number one health threat."[1]

My most recent forays into losing weight have been Entering The
Zone and then most recently Dr. Atkins creation where I lived on
bacon and eggs, steaks, fish, cheese and chicken with a salad a day.
Though I did lose half my initial goal of 40 pounds in 4 months the
last 20 pounds hardly budged. As I continued that way of eating
into my fifth month, I realized between all the meat and the Atkins
low carb products, I was spending a small fortune. I couldn't escape
the nagging feeling this kind of eating caused and I knew it couldn't
be good for me over the long haul. Between my understanding the
theory of "you are what you eat" and my intuition whispering in
my ear "you're killing yourself," I got my answer loud and clear
from an unusual direction. All my life I have been blessed with
never needing to use deodorant, but once the odor of all that

---
[1] USA Today and front page comcast website June 11, 2003

decaying flesh in my system started to make its presence known, I knew this wasn't something I could do for life.

Fortunately, someone did figure out a better way 2000 years ago. Unfortunately, it has taken nineteen plus centuries to reach the surface. The fact is, this diet is about as simple as it gets and the results (even if you cheat) are amazing. This way of living not only sheds the pounds, but heals your body as well, while making you look and feel years younger. I didn't create this diet plan. It's wisdom of the ages and I'm just the messenger. I will promise you this much if you embrace this simple way of living. It will:

1. Give you more energy than you've probably ever known.
2. Help you find your natural body weight where all your favorite clothes fit once again.
3. Bring on a peace of mind and clarity of thought you probably never knew existed.
4. Eliminate any and all unpleasant body odor from your breath to your pores.
5. Clear up various allergies, many aches and pains, and help you to live the long life humans are meant to enjoy.
6. Increase your sexual stamina. (Actually neither Jesus or Szekely put it quite like that, I added number six to make sure I had your attention.)

These are just a few of the outcomes you can expect from this way of living. The fact is, if I told you all of what Jesus claimed would be the result of this way of living, you wouldn't believe me anyway. For all you 'Doubting Thomas' out there who have tried every diet fad that has come along, Szekely was testing this diet long before any of them were written and collected. There are more than 50 years of data, complete with numerous before and after photos for your viewing pleasure. There's one amazing story you can find in Szekely's "Search For The Ageless Vol.1" that is dramatic proof of how this diet can heal your body as well as the other claims I made above.

After first discovering this treasure trove of information, Szekely decided to put it to the test. He took the Essene method of healing that Jesus had described and set off to heal a leper colony in Tahiti.

There he either cured or put into remission every single patient in
the colony. As Szekely wrote later, we were "spectacularly
successful in improving the condition and even curing it."[2] Szekely
then moved to Mexico and opened a health clinic where he
conducted what he called The Great Experiment, treating 123,600
people over a 33 year period with this same diet and health
program advocated by Jesus. Of the 123,000 plus who came to his
clinic, approximately 17% of the clients showed up with the
medical diagnosis of "incurable." Of the entire 123, 600 people,
90% *regained full health,* including many of the supposedly
incurables.[3]

   When you consider that Szekely practiced it on well over a
hundred thousand people on five continents over half a dozen
decades with tremendous success, I'd say you have a fairly
thorough track record to follow. Folks, this isn't some pie in the sky
scheme I've made up to set your hopes up one more time. It really
does work. My hope is to inspire you to go to the source and see
for yourself. Towards that end I'll later refer you to many of
Szekely's 80 plus books that he wrote about his findings.

   So dig in, or as my grandfather used to say when we'd sit down
to eat, "grab a root and growl." If you should perchance decide to
live what you read, you'll get not only the physical blessings I've
described, but the mental, emotional and spiritual blessings as well.
If not totally convinced in 90 days, we'll gladly refund your misery.
(And no, Jesus didn't say that either.) It comes from knowing and
not simply believing this to be truth. Like Szekely before me, I put
it to the test by using myself as the guinea pig.

---

[2] Edmond Bordeaux Szekely "Search for the Ageless, Vol One," 98-118, International
   Biogenic Society
[3] International Biogenic Society

The Basic Diet
in The Words Of Jesus

"The greatness of a nation can be judged by the way its animals
are treated."   *– Mahatma Gandhi*

"And it was by the bed of a stream many sick fasted and prayed
with God's angels (sun, air, water) for seven days and seven
nights. And great was their reward, for they followed Jesus
words. And with the passing of the seventh day, all their pains left
them. And when the sun rose over the earth's rim they saw Jesus
coming towards them from the mountain with the brightness of
the rising sun about his head."

"Peace be with you."[1]

And they said no word at all but cast themselves before him, and
touched the hem of his garment in token of their healing.

"Give thanks not to me, but to your earthly mother who sent
you her healing angels. Go and sin no more, that you may never
see disease. And let the healing angels become your guardians."

But they answered him: "Tell us, what are the sins from which we
must shun, that we may nevermore see disease?" Jesus answered:
"Be it so according to your faith," and he sat down among them
saying:

"It was said to them of old time: 'Honor thy Heavenly Father
and thy Earthly Mother, and do their commandments that thy
days may be long upon the earth… And next afterward was given
the commandment, 'Thou shall not kill' for life is given to all by

---

[1] The Discovery of the Essene Gospel of Peace, Edmund Bordeaux Szekely, International
Biogenic Society

God, and that which God has given, let not man take away. For I
tell you truly, from one mother proceeds all that lives upon the
earth. Therefore, he who kills, kills his brother and from him will
the Earthly Mother turn away…and he will be shunned by her
angels……and the flesh of slain beasts in his body will become his
own tomb. For I tell you truly, he who kills, kills himself, and
those who eat flesh of slain beasts, eats of the body of death. For
in his blood, every drop of their blood turns to poison; in his
breath, their breath to stink; in his flesh their flesh to boils; in his
bones their bones to chalk; in his bowels their bowels to decay, in
his eyes their eyes to scales; in his ears their ears to waxy issue;
and their dead will become his dead."

"Kill not, neither eat the flesh of your innocent prey, lest you
become the slave of evil. For that is the path of sufferings and
leads unto death."

"But do the will of God that his angels will serve you on the
way of life. Obey, therefore, the words of God: 'Behold I have
given you every herb bearing seed, which is upon the face of all
the earth, and every tree, in which is the fruit of a tree yielding
seed; to you it shall be for meat. I give every green herb for meat.
Also the milk of everything that moveth and that liveth upon the
earth shall be meat for you.…But flesh, and the blood that
quickens it, shall ye
not eat.'

"For I tell you truly, man is more than the beast. But he who
kills a beast without a cause, though the beast attack him not,
through lust for slaughter, or for its flesh, or for its hide, or even
its tusks, evil is the deed which he does, for he is turned into a
wild beast himself."[2]

OK, that seems pretty clear. Don't eat meat, as once it's inside of
you it starts to turn your body into a tomb. Hmm – that might even
have to be considered the exact opposite of treating your body like
a temple. If that's not enough, think about the smell of decaying
flesh that eventually has to come out of your pores. One vegetarian
friend of mine 30 years ago used to make fun of my eating habits
when we'd go out to eat by asking the waitress for "a dead cow and

---

[2] Szekely "The Essene Origins of Christianity"

a glass of blood please." Unfortunately I wasn't ready to hear that wisdom and ordered either a cow or a chicken or a pig served up.

Then another said: "Moses the greatest in Israel, suffered our forefathers to eat the flesh of clean beasts, and forbade only the flesh of unclean beasts. Why therefore do you forbid us the flesh of all beasts? Which law comes from God? That of Moses or your law?" And Jesus answered them:

"God gave, by Moses, the commandments to your forefathers. 'These commandments are hard,' said your forefathers and could not keep them. When Moses saw this, he had compassion on his people, and would not that they perish. And then he gave them 10 times 10 commandments, less hard, that they might follow them. I tell you truly, if your forefathers had been able to keep the 10 commandments of God, Moses would never have had need of the 10 times 10 commandments...and of these ten times ten the scribes and Pharisees have made a hundred times ten commandments. And they have unbearable burdens upon your shoulders, that they themselves do not carry. For the more nigh are the commandments of God, the less do we need; and the further they are from God, then the more do we need. Wherefore are the laws of the Scribes and Pharisees innumerable; the laws of the son of man seven; of the angels three; and of God one."[3]

Looks to me like his wisdom is directed at anyone who might want to rationalize their killing of animals and eating flesh from Old Testament verses, so he reminds them that "thou shall not kill" was meant for everything living not just other men. He makes this point even clearer a little further along.

And all were astonished at his wisdom, and asked him: "Continue master and teach us all the laws which we can receive." And Jesus continued:

"God commanded your forefathers, 'Thou shall not kill.' But their heart was hardened and they killed. Then Moses desired that at least they should not kill men, and he suffered them to kill beasts. And then the heart of your forefathers was hardened yet more, and they killed men and beasts likewise. But I say unto you:

---

[3] The Discovery of the Essene Gospel of Peace, Edmund Bordeaux Szekely, International Biogenic Society

Kill neither man, nor beasts, nor yet the food which goes into your mouth. For if you eat living food, the same will quicken you, but if you kill your food, the dead food will kill you also. For life always comes from life, and from death comes always death. For everything which kills your foods, kills your bodies also. And everything that kills your bodies kills your souls also. And your bodies become what your foods are, even as your spirits likewise become what your thoughts are. You shall live only by the fire of life, and prepare not your foods with the fire of death, which kills your foods, your bodies and your souls also..."

Later, when Jesus is speaking of the animals he said, "And whatsoever ye do unto the least of these my children (the animals), ye do it unto me. For I am in them, and they are in me. In all their joys I rejoice, in all their afflictions I am afflicted. Wherefore I say unto all who desire to be my disciples, keep your hands from bloodshed and let no flesh meat enter your mouths."

It makes perfect sense that Moses would relax the rules on killing animals to try and get his people to at least not kill other men. How many times have we all heard "you are what you eat" and never gave it a second thought. It seems there might be something to it after all. And then to hear that our spirits become what our thoughts are focused upon really starts to make sense.

"Master, where is the fire of life?" asked some of them.

"In you, in your blood and in your bodies."

"And the fire of death?" asked others.

"It is the fire that blazes outside your body, which is hotter than your blood. With that fire of death you cook your foods in your homes and in your fields. I tell you truly, it is the same fire which destroys your foods and your bodies, even as the law of malice, which ravages your thoughts, and ravages your spirits."

"For your body is that which you eat, and your spirit is that which you think. Eat nothing therefore which a stronger fire than the fire of life has killed. Wherefore prepare and eat all fruits and trees, and all grasses of the fields, and all milk of beasts good for eating. For all these are fed and ripened by the fire of life (the sun), all are the gifts of the angels of our earthly mother. But eat nothing to which only the fire of death gives savor."

"So eat always from the table of God: the fruits of the trees, the grain of the grasses of the field, the milk of beasts, and the honey of bees. For everything beyond these leads by the way of diseases unto death. But the foods which you eat from the abundant table of God give strength and youth to your body, and you will never see disease. For the table of God fed Methuselah of old, and I tell you truly, if you live even as he lived, then will the God of the living give you also long life upon the earth as was his."[4]

One of the most interesting aspects to me is how he knew that cooking foods would kill their nutrition value, as this only became a known scientific fact in the second half of the 20th century. Most people prefer their vegetables cooked, though thanks to my earthly father I've known that eating foods picked right off the vine was a delight since I was just a young boy. I also loved the analogy of how the fire we used to cook our foods at home would ruin our bodies much the same way malice would ravage our thoughts and spirits. There are numerous other verses like this where Jesus says it in other ways, but I think he makes his point pretty clear on what he thinks we should be eating and what we should leave well enough alone.

The Basic Diet Rules
The 10 Commandments

1 "Eat all things even as they are found on the table of the earthly mother. Cook not, neither mix all things one with the another, lest your bowels become as steaming bogs...be content with two or three sorts of foods which you will always find on the table of your earthly mother. And desire not to devour all things which you see around you. For I tell you truly, if you mix together all sorts of food in your body, then the peace of your body will cease, and endless war will rage in you."

Modern English Version: Eat only raw foods (fruits, vegetables, grains, dairy products and honey) and eat them when they are as fresh as possible. Neither cook them or mix them up with other foods as your stomach works best that has to work least. It's

---

[4] Everything in this section comes from "The Essene Origins of Christianity."

obvious Jesus recommended a natural food diet as best. Keep it
simple. Only eat two or three different items at a meal whenever
possible.

Real world findings: Living on fruits, nuts and vegetables is a lot
easier than you would think. There are dozens of books with
delicious vegetarian recipe and juice cocktails to keep you from
getting bored. The problem with bread can become a bit sticky but
Jesus even gives us a recipe later for making bread that sprouts in
the sun and doesn't need to be baked at all or go to your local
health food store and try some "Manna Bread." With our fast
paced world I recommend not getting too fanatical at first though
you might think about changing your pace a bit as well. Don't beat
yourself up if at first you slip now and then! When it comes to
cooking with the sun, it can be fun but Jesus lived in a desert so it
would have been a lot easier back then. You can always use a food
dehydrator that will accomplish the task. The reason for all this
trouble is that the living enzymes of the wheat are essential to a
healthy body, but are destroyed when cooked at a temperature of
118 degrees or higher. This is true of all food cooked over 118
degrees, as temperatures higher than this will destroy the enzymes.
Jesus knew this 2,000 years ago and our modern science has now
proven it to be true. I've included more about the importance of
enzymes in a later chapter. As to eating only two or three different
foods at a time, this one I have found a bit difficult so I have bent
that rule allowing myself four or five instead.

2 "And when you eat, never eat unto fullness. Flee the
temptations and listen to the voice of God's angels. You will
always be tempted to eat more and more, but live by the
spirit and resist the desires of the body. And your fasting is
always pleasing in the eyes of the angels of God. So give heed
to how much you have eaten when your body is sated, and
always eat less by a third."

Modern English Version: Never eat until you feel full and pay
attention to your body's own signals. Your body doesn't require
near as much food as you think it does and will work at its

optimum peak if you follow this advice. I've found the weekly one day fast (rule #9) makes this much easier than I first imagined it would be.

Real World Findings: Once you start fasting, eating slower, and chewing up your food better, this will get a lot easier as your body was designed to give clear signals. Though modern man has effectively drowned them out, they will return usually within the first two weeks of this diet.

3 "For I tell you truly, he who eats more than twice in the day does in him the work of Satan…. Eat only when the sun is highest in the heavens, and again when it is set, and you will never see disease. The angels will rejoice in your body, and your days will be long upon the earth, for this is pleasing in the eyes of the Lord."

Modern English Version: Contrary to many modern diets, Jesus recommends not eating so often. Your body needs down time when it's not digesting food to repair other systems. (I'll go into more scientific details later.) He tells us it's preferable to eat at noon and then again around sunset. Since they didn't have the modern convenience of electric light back then I imagine they went to bed a good bit earlier than modern man, so feel free to bend this one a bit on the evening side, but try not to break bread 'til noon.

Real World Findings: I call this the 'no breakfast clause' as it is a continuation of your nightly fast. In the numerous pages Jesus talks about diet, fasting is easily the thing he stresses most often and for numerous reasons. My experience has been that most people (coffee addicts excepted) find this a lot easier than you'd think after the first 2 weeks. Many have felt that the mental clarity alone was worth the price of admission.

4 "Eat not unclean foods brought from far countries, but eat always that which your trees bear. For your God knows well what is needful for you and where and when. And he gives to all peoples of all kingdoms for food that which is best for each."

Modern English Version: Eat foods that are local to your area whenever possible. Keep to a minimum all foods that have to be shipped in from far away.

Real World Findings: If you have a local produce stand where you can go, or can find local gardens and local orchards to get your fruits and vegetables, that is the ideal. A lot more health food stores are starting to carry this kind of home-grown produce. Personally, I love Thai food and Indian food but try and eat them only on special occasions now that I see the results of this advice. Not only am I eating food and spices that are foreign to my natural environment but it is usually served hot. Also when I do go to exotic restaurants I try and eat mostly the cold dishes now. It's a small price to pay for my health. Also, when your local foods are in season, buy extra and freeze them or dry them with a dehydrator as they keep most of their nutrient value that way as well.

5   "Eat not as heathens do, who stuff themselves in haste, defiling their bodies with all manners of abominations. For the power of God's angels enters into you with the living food which the Lord gives you from his royal table."

Modern English Version: Slow down when you eat and even take notice of what starts to occur when you put living (as opposed to dead) food in your body. Though music and social intercourse were very much a part of their lives back then, there are innumerable passages that mention how mealtimes were done in ritual and quiet reflection.

Real World Findings: This might be the most difficult of all the admonitions as the terms "fast food" and "drive through" suggest. We have been so inculcated with the idea that it is a modern convenience to have speedy meals and snacks to pick us up throughout the day, we don't even notice we often eat out of sheer habit and not hunger at all. Slowing down and being conscious of one's actions goes contrary to the pace life has become in the 21st century . For that reason alone, it should maybe become a priority to wait until you can slow down and give your temple the attention it deserves before you break your fast.

6 "Breathe long and deeply at all your meals that the angel of air may bless your repasts. And chew well your food with your teeth, that it becomes water and that angel of water turn it into blood in your body. And eat slowly as it were a prayer you make to the Lord. For I tell you truly, the power of God enters into you if you eat after this manner at his table. For the table of the Lord is as an altar, and he who eats at the table of God, is in a temple."

Modern English Version: Breathing deep and chewing well are obviously very important activities when one breaks bread. It's as important how you eat as is what you eat. From a strictly weight loss perspective you will feel full much quicker when you chew your food more and this will naturally cause you to eat less. From a health perspective, it gets the natural digestive enzymes into your bloodstream quicker and easier. From a spiritual perspective this becomes prayer time so even if you don't talk to God any other time, you're reminded to do it here.

Real World Findings: Depends on the individual. It gets easier with practice so you might try practicing this type of eating alone at first as it is very difficult when breaking bread with others who aren't on the same path. Just like working out at the gym, it's much easier in the beginning to have a work-out partner so maybe think about finding a diet partner you can practice this intentional way of eating with. Not chewing well causes your enzymes (that would ordinarily be working on repairing other parts of your body), to have to give all their attention to digesting your food. So if you're eating constantly and not chewing your food well, the system designed to keep you in health has no choice but to take its attention away from areas that might be needing it just so you can digest your food.

7 "For I tell you truly, the body of the Sons of Man is turned into a temple, and their inwards into an altar, if you do the commandments of God. Wherefore, put naught upon the altar of the Lord when your spirit is vexed, neither think upon anyone with anger in the temple of God. Enter into the

Lord's sanctuary when you feel in yourselves the call of his
angels, for all that you eat in sorrow, or in anger, or without
desire, becomes a poison in your body...and let all evil
thoughts depart from you when you receive into your body
the power of God from his table."

Modern English Version: Don't even set the table or think about
breaking bread when you are angry as it will turn to poison within
you. The power of one's thought will affect you on levels most of
us aren't even aware. Try to clear your mind and be at peace when
you go to eat. When you eat from habit instead of hunger you're
poisoning yourself.

Real World Findings: This one can be difficult as well but will get
easier as you set your intentions to follow it. Try to do a mental
gratitude list to change your mood if you're hungry and irritable at
the same time – if not successful, it's better to fast than to poison
yourself. Many of us use food to stuff our feelings down which is
likely the biggest cause of obesity in the world. This one
admonition alone, if followed religiously *(no pun intended),* can
change your life.

8 "Never sit at the table of God before he calls you by the angel
of appetite...and your life will be long upon the earth, for the
most precious of God's servants will serve you all your days:
the angel of joy."

Modern English Version: Again we see stressed the importance of
not eating for any reason except when our body truly needs
nourishment. The reward will be a long and joyful life.

Real World Findings: Most often we eat to kill time, to keep our
hands busy, to stuff uncomfortable feelings, to be sociable, to please
grandma, because a TV commercial comes on, or because three
meals a day is the way your parents and their parents did it. Clean
your plate, think about all the starving children in Ethiopia. You
don't get desert till you've eaten all your spinach! Many of us eat
whether we're hungry or not strictly out of habit. If you want the
best life has to offer it's time to *break the habit!*

9 "Forget not that every seventh day is holy and consecrated to God. On six days feed your body with the gifts of the earthly mother, but on the seventh day sanctify your body for your Heavenly Father. And on the seventh day eat not of earthly foods, but live only upon the words of God."

Modern English Version: Fast one day a week. Abstain from any food for an entire day while allowing your focus to turn to more spiritual pursuits. Even in the biblical 'canon,' fasting is mentioned 74 times. Jesus did it regularly as did all his disciples. Many people lose three or four pounds a day at the beginning of a fast and then level off to a pound a day after they've purified their body awhile. Granted, much of this is water weight, but it sure feels good psychologically to see yourself 15-20 pounds lighter on the scale than you were just a week before. Also, contrary to what you might have heard in the past, fasting is the healthiest thing you can do for your body. Few people realize that humans are the only sentient beings that don't fast when they get ill. Every animal in nature does it as it is nature's way of healing the body. Unfortunately, we've been taught you have to eat to keep up your strength, when in actuality that often isn't the case at all, as one will discover the first time they do an extended fast.

Real World Findings: The first one day fast might feel a bit uncomfortable but this too shall pass. This is probably the most important key to being successful on this diet. *Don't skip this one as it makes all the other rules so much easier.* Whereas other diets tell you it's OK to binge one day a week, Jesus and the Essenes say just the opposite. Fasting just one day a week seems to unlock the doors of many of the other admonitions and makes them all that much easier to incorporate into one's life. For the secular minded reader consider spending intimate time with your children or going out for a walk in nature, or even sitting outdoors (when weather permits) reading a book. A day spent leaning against a tree can work miracles! When it comes to fasting, start slowly, sticking to juice fasts for the first few times until you've cleaned out some of your life-long toxic buildup. I guarantee it's there. Eventually you can move up to water fasts, the results of which will amaze you.

My first long water fast I lost 15 pounds in the first six days alone.
If you're too thin already, don't worry, when you break the fast
with healthy foods, you will naturally return to your correct body
weight quite rapidly. Only this time you're rebuilding your body
with healthy cells. Look up fasting on the web. Arnold Ehret's
"Mucousless Diet," which has much information about fasting, was
written in the early 1900's and healed thousands of people.

10 "And God will send you each morning the angel of
sunshine to wake you from your sleep. Therefore, obey
your summons and lie not idle in your beds for the angels
of air and water await you already…But when the sun sets
and the Heavenly Father sends you his most precious angel,
sleep, then take your rest, and be all night with the angel of
sleep that his unknown angels may be with you the lifelong
night … and they will teach you many things concerning
the kingdom of God, even as the angels that you know of
the Earthly Mother (sun, water, air) instruct you in the
things of her kingdom. For I tell you truly, you will be
every night the guests of the kingdom of your Heavenly
Father, if you do his commandments. And when you wake
upon the morrow, you will feel in you the power of the
unknown angels. Your Heavenly Father will send them to
you every night, that they may build your spirit even as
every day the Earthly Mother sends you angels that they
may build your body. For I tell you truly, if in the daytime
your Earthly Mother folds you in her arms, and in the
night the Heavenly Father breathes his kiss upon you, they
will The Sons of Men become the Sons of God."

Modern English Version: Give more significance to the
importance of sleep, as it is the most precious angel of all. Going
into a good sleep is how we invite what he calls "the unknown
angels" in to do their work. We should consider sleep as an
invitation to the divine, so that when you awaken, you will be filled
with the power given by your angels in your dreams.

Real World Findings: Many of us tend to take sleep for granted when it is obviously a very important part of our day though on a level most of us don't understand. I try and express gratitude and then give my angels (my subconscious mind) jobs to do before drifting off each night. It's amazing how many problems can be solved while you sleep.

These are the 10 basic rules to have the weight loss and energy enhancing promises come true. I've found that even if you decide to only follow a few of them completely, such as stopping the meat and fasting once a week, you will still see dramatic results. We'll come back to specific food combinations and the scientific reasoning behind them later, but for now I'd like to take you on a tour of the grounds on which this program is built. This next section is geared more towards the physical healing, the mental and emotional clarity, and the spiritual connection which Jesus says is available to everyone once they have cleansed the body through fasting and proper diet. For a more rewarding, joy filled life, I highly recommend adopting at least some of what I refer to as the "wake-up call" part of the program.

Wake-up Call

"Nothing will benefit human health and increase the chances for survival on earth as much as the evolution to a vegetarian diet."
– Albert Einstein

Enhanced health is only one reason Jesus advocated the raw food diet. His primary motivation was a spiritual one, based on the ethic of compassion as illustrated in the following passage:[1]

Jesus, speaking of animals said, "And whatsoever ye do unto these the least of my children (the animals), ye do unto me. For I am in them, and they are in me. In all their joys I rejoice, in all their afflictions I am afflicted. Wherefore I say unto all who desire to be my disciples, keep your hands from bloodshed and let no flesh meat enter your mouths." Later on he adds, "Verily I say unto you, they who partake of benefits which are gotten by wronging one of God's creatures, cannot be righteous: nor can they understand holy things, or teach the mysteries of the kingdom, whose hands are stained with blood or whose mouths are defiled with flesh…"

Though it is quite clear that Jesus only required his new disciples to practice basic vegetarianism, he strongly urged his veteran disciples to go even further as he describes himself as a fruitarian:

"For of the fruits of the trees and the seeds of the earth alone do I partake, and these are changed by the spirit into my flesh and my blood. Of these alone and their like shall ye eat who believe in me, and are my disciples, for of these, in the spirit, come life and health and healing unto man…..God giveth the grains and the

---

[1] Szekely, Edmond Bordeaux, "The Essene New Testament"

fruits of the earth: and for righteous man truly there is no other lawful sustenance for the body."[2]

"A disciple of Jesus asked him a question, saying, 'Master, if there come to us any that eat flesh... shall we receive them?"

"And Jesus said unto him, let such abide in the outer court till they cleanse themselves from these grosser evils; for till they perceive, and repent of these, they are not fit to receive the higher mysteries."

Modern English Version: Seems pretty clear that he's admonishing those that would pursue the spiritual path that they must first learn to treat the body as a temple. This even sounds like a prerequisite before they are ready for his deeper teachings.

"There is none yet among you that can understand all of this of which I speak. He who expounds to you the scriptures speaks to you in a dead tongue of dead men, through his diseased and mortal body. Him therefore, can all men understand, for all men are diseased and all are in death. Blind man leads blind on the dark paths of disease and suffering....I have still many things to say to you, but you cannot hear them yet. For your eyes are used to the darkness and the full light of the Heavenly Father would make you blind. Therefore you cannot yet understand that which I speak to you of the Heavenly Father who sent me to you. Follow therefore first, only the laws of your Earthly Mother, of which I have told you. And when her angels (air, water and sun) shall have cleansed and renewed your bodies and strengthened your eyes, you will be able to bear the light of our Heavenly Father. When you can gaze on the brightness of the noon day sun with unflinching eyes, you can then look upon the blinding light of your Heavenly Father."

Modern English Version: First and foremost we must clean out our temples by fasting, breathing fresh air, drinking clean water and basking daily in the rays of the sun!

After reading the last line of that passage about gazing on the noon day sun I remembered the most amazing story I need to relate that happened to me over two decades earlier.

I had become friends with a man I had met at my home church

---

[2] Ibid

(The Hiding Place in Los Angeles) who undoubtedly had the most magnificent eyes of any human I have ever encountered. His name was Jules Bucchieri and he lived in the Bel Air section of Los Angeles. Jules was an entrepreneur, musician and spiritual adept who had once managed Lenny Bruce and owned the property on which the famous Morton's Restaurant was built in Beverly Hills. Jules had been into pure foods as far back as the 60's, and relished serving vegetarian feasts at his home to people from all walks of life. He seemed to know everyone in LA and was a true delight to all who knew him.

One weekend he invited me to drive with him up the coast of California where we were both going to participate in Johnny River's (Secret Agent Man) wedding. I'll never forget that ceremony as it was outdoors on the cliffs overlooking the ocean in Big Sur, and the 'bride to be' came riding up in a horse drawn carriage while young maidens dropped rose petals all along the path. I played some of the wedding music that day and remember the exquisite timing of a whale breaching the surface below just as Johnny and his bride were saying "I do!"

But what stands out to me even more was a conversation I had with Jules on the way back down the coast when I asked him why his eyes were so magnificently beautiful, unlike anything I had ever seen. Not just the color, mind you, but they literally seemed to sparkle with life. He then told me how they had once been a very ordinary brown and that he even had to wear corrective lens. He continued on and showed me the practice he had been taught which had changed them to the exquisite gaze I saw before me. Now, after reading that last statement by Jesus about gazing at the noon day sun I think it is time to share Jules' secret with the world.

He told me he made a point to never wear sunglasses and daily practiced gazing towards the sun. "For starters", he said, "I only did it when the sun was less severe and I would move my fingers rapidly back and forth in front of my eyes to block out the harshest rays." In time though, he told me, he was able to actually gaze directly upon the sun and in so doing he had eventually healed his vision as well as changed their color from brown to the indescribable hue that I saw before me that day. Remembering this, after reading the words of Jesus, I decided to be my own guinea pig and started practicing Jules technique. Here are the results:

After six weeks of practice I could no longer read using just my current contact lenses, and had to put on reading glasses to use with them. Within a few more days even with the reading glasses I was finding it difficult to read. So I took out my contacts to use my regular glasses and my eyes hurt so badly I had to take the glasses off immediately. I knew then, it wasn't my imagination – my eyes were either a lot better or a lot worse, so I went to an optometrist in Ann Arbor, Michigan for a full eye exam. I need to preface this by telling you in my 25 years of wearing contact lenses, the six or eight changes I've made over the years have always been because my eyes were progressively worse and a stronger prescription was always needed. The optometrist was amazed as he wrote out the new prescription as my vision had improved dramatically. I decided then not to incur the expense of new glasses till I saw how far this would go. To make a long story short, I had to go back to the optometrist again two weeks later and had to get yet another prescription as my eyes had improved even more. Unfortunately, not being a scientist, and not really expecting the results to be so dramatic, I didn't think to conduct this experiment in a controlled environment and had begun another experiment, a short water fast, almost at the beginning of my eye experiment. That short water fast stretched into 36 days with no food and became much more of a priority than paying attention to my eyes. Upon resuming my normal diet my eyes again returned to their previous prescription. Conclusions: none at this point, though it sure amazed my optometrist when I kept showing up needing weaker and weaker prescriptions. (After the second time in less than a month that he had to revise my prescription, I told him that I might need to get an affidavit as I was planning on telling the story in a book.)

"All those around him listened with amazement for his word was with power, and taught quite otherwise than the priests and scribes. And thought the sun was now set, they departed not for their homes. They sat around about Jesus and asked him: 'Master, which are these laws of life? Rest with us awhile and teach us.'" And Jesus answered:

"Seek not the law in your scriptures, for the law is life, whereas the scripture is dead. I tell you truly, Moses received not his laws from God in writing, but through his living word. The law is living word of living God to living prophets for living men. In everything that is life is the law written. You find it in the grass, in the tree, in the river, in the mountain, in the birds of heaven, in the fishes of the sea, but seek it chiefly in yourselves. For I tell you truly, all living things are nearer to God than the scriptures which are without life. God so made life and all living things that they might be the everlasting word teaching the laws of the true God to man. God wrote not the laws in the pages of books, but in your heart and in your spirit. They are in your breath, your blood, your bones, your flesh, your bowels, your eyes, your ears and every little part of your body. They are present in the air, in the earth, in the plants, in the sunbeams, in the depths and in the heights. They all speak to you that you may understand the tongue and the will of the living God. But you shut your eyes that you may not see, and you shut your ears that you may not hear. I tell you truly, that the scripture is the work of man, but life and all its hosts are the work of God. Wherefore (why) do you not listen to the words of God which are written in his works? And wherefore (why) do you study the dead scriptures which are the works of the hands of men?"

Modern English Version: Everything that has life is where we should find our answers to life. God speaks to us through his creations and especially though ourselves if we will just go within and listen. "All living things" he says "are nearer to God than the scriptures which are without life." In the very first line he sums it up when he says to not look for the law in any books "For the law is life, whereas the scripture is dead."

Real World Findings: Not a whole lot of wiggle room there that I can see, but in case you need a bit more clarification, Jesus continued on:

"You do not understand the words of life because you are in death. For I tell you, it profits you not at all that you pore over the dead scriptures if by your deeds you deny him who has given you the scriptures. If you will that the living God's word and his power may enter you, defile not your body, for your body is the temple of the spirit, and the spirit is the temple of God. Purify therefore the temple that the Lord of the temple may dwell therein and occupy a place that is worthy of him."

"Renew yourselves and fast. For I tell you truly, that Satan and his plagues may only be cast out by fasting and prayer. Go by yourself and fast alone, and show your fasting to no man."

Modern English Version: He says most people don't understand his teachings because they themselves are dead from spending their time poring over scriptures that are also dead. He goes on to say if you want the many blessings that he has promised us, we must first purify the body itself, as that is the temple and we must make it worthy of God before he will enter. Once again he reiterates on the importance of fasting and prayer. Also, for the first time that I've encountered he talks about the importance of fasting alone.

Real World Findings: He's quite adamant that if you truly want "the living God's word and his power" then only through fasting and prayer or by following the practices of Jesus' DieT will you get there.

How to Reap the Benefits of Health and Clarity

1. "Seek the fresh air of the forest and of all the fields, and there in the midst of them shall you find the angel of air. Put off your shoes and your clothing and suffer the angel of air to embrace all your body. Then breathe long and deeply, that the angel of air may be brought within you. The angel of air shall cast out of your body all uncleanness which defiled it without and within you. And thus shall all evil smelling and unclean things rise out of you, as the smoke of fire curls upwards and is lost in the sea of the air. For I tell you truly, holy is the angel of the air, who cleanses all that is unclean and makes all evil-smelling things of a sweet odor. No man may come before the face of God whom the angel of air lets not pass."

Modern English Version: Breathe, Breathe, Breathe. Seek out locations in nature where you can take off your shoes and discard your clothing and practice deep breathing while being "embraced" by the "angel of air."

Real World Findings: Otherwise known as prana. There's nothing quite so healing as a good yoga class. Find a style of yoga that suits you (there are many westernized versions available) and an instructor that will work with you at your own level. I guarantee you'll be glad you did. Put signs up all over your house reminding yourself to take long, deep breaths.

2. "After the angel of air, seek the angel of water. Put off your shoes and your clothing and suffer the angel of water to embrace all your body. The angel of water shall cast out of your body all uncleanness which defiled it without and within you just as the uncleannesses of the garments washed in water flow away and are lost in the stream of the river. For I tell you truly, holy is the angel of the water, who cleanses all that is unclean and makes all evil-smelling things of a sweet odor. No man may come before the face of God whom the angel of water lets not pass. In very truth, all must be born again of water and of truth, for your body bathes in the river of earthly life, and your spirit bathes in the river of life everlasting. For you receive your blood from our Earthly Mother and the truth from our Heavenly Father."

Modern English Version: Water, agua, H_2O. Swim in it, float on it, drink lots of it, and then drink some more. This should be done especially out in nature where you can take off your shoes and discard your clothing and immerse yourself while being "embraced" by the "angel of water." So there is a reason many health spas have a cold water dip.

Real World Findings: From the dieter's point of view, water is your best friend. Un-carbonated, natural water in your system at all times. Carry it with you always and treat it with reverence as it is one of your best friends. When Szekely was busy healing the lepers in Tahiti he had them moving in and through the water daily. He called it "compulsory water ballet."

3. "And if afterward there remains within you any of your past sins and uncleannesses, seek the angel of sunlight. Put off your shoes and your clothing and suffer the angel of sunlight to embrace all your body. Then breathe long and deeply, that

the angel of sunlight may be brought within you. And the angel of sunlight shall cast out of your body all evil smelling and unclean things which defiled it without and within. For I tell you truly, holy is the angel of the sunlight, who cleanses all uncleannesses and makes all evil-smelling things of a sweet odor. None may come before the face of God, whom the angel of water lets not pass. Truly, all must be born again of sun and of truth, for your body basks in the sunlight of Earthly Mother, and your spirit basks in the sunlight of truth from your Heavenly Father."

Modern English Version: Bask in the sunlight as much as you can. Seek out locations in nature where you can take off your shoes and discard your clothing, and practice basking under, and breathing in, the rays of light while being "embraced" by the "angel of sunshine."

Real World Findings: A word of caution here as mankind has destroyed much of our ozone layer since the days when Jesus walked about. Also if you're fair skinned, you need to remember that people in that region of the world had dark complexions back then. Use natural sun-blocks on the skin and choose your times to bask in sunlight, carefully avoiding the most intense rays in the middle of the day. Practice the sun gazing technique I described as well, but again avoid the most intense sun as you experiment with this technique.

Jesus continued on:

"The angels of air and water and of sunlight are brethren. They were given to The Son of Man that they might serve him, and that he might go always from one to the other. Holy is their embrace. They are indivisible children of the Earthly Mother, so do not you put asunder those whom heaven and earth have made one. Let these three brothers angels enfold you every day and let them abide with you through all your fasting."

"Follow the example of the running water, the wind as it blows, the rising and setting of the sun, the growing plants and trees, the beasts as they run and gamble, the wane and waxing of the moon, the starts as they come and go again; all these do move and perform their labors. For all which has life does move, and only that which is dead is still."

"It was said to you: 'Honor thy father and thy mother that thy days may be long upon this earth.' But I say to you Sons of Man: Honor your Earthly Mother and keep all her laws, that your days may be long on this earth, and honor your Heavenly Father that eternal life may be yours in the heavens. For the Heavenly Father is a hundred times greater than all fathers by seed and by blood, and greater is the Earthly Mother than all mothers by the body….and your true brothers are all those who do the will of your Heavenly Father and your Earthly Mother and not your brothers by blood."

Summation

"The doctor of the future will give no medicine, but will interest his patients in the cure of the human frame in diet, and in the cause and prevention of disease."
— *Thomas A. Edison*

I've purposely taken a lot of time to establish not only the common sense but the foundation of where this diet originated. Only once I was convinced this was the diet of Jesus himself, was I willing to really go for it. Stopping meat all together felt like a big decision and one that I wouldn't try without some serious motivation. Once I was convinced this was truly the answer to "what would Jesus eat?" I knew I was ready to give it a go.

I was raised in a Baptist family and saw more than my share of potluck meals and the kinds of foods that were typically served. It's become my belief that many of the fattest people in the world and especially in America are the dedicated Christians, and it dawned on me that even if they wouldn't listen to their doctors they might be willing to listen to the words of Jesus. I'd love to see someone do a study on the correlation between obesity and organized religion, especially Christianity. I'm also convinced that our fast paced lifestyles and eating habits are clearly behind the epidemic of heart problems, cancer and many other modern ailments. So many people are hooked on fast food that it has clearly become responsible for a big part of that epidemic. Even when people do take the time to eat a healthy meal, they often stuff the food in their mouths and swallow without barely chewing, thereby getting negligible nutrition that the body requires. Add all that up with our national habit of eating while we sit in front of a TV, watching images that poison our thoughts, and it's no wonder we're in a crisis. I figured if people (Christian and non-Christian alike) could learn how to follow the example that Jesus set with foods that are available today, they might realize the health benefits of the food Jesus ate while avoiding so many modern health risks.

For the Christian reader out there, the market is flooded with diet programs, each claiming to be the solution to a healthy lifestyle. While some of them might be based on biblical principles, there is no other program that truthfully answers the question what would Jesus do, or better yet, what would Jesus eat? Not only was Jesus himself adamant on the subject of diet, as we've discovered in the Essene texts, but the rewards of this diet were known even back in the times of the Old Testament, as shown by what has been called the 'Daniel challenge.'

For those of you not familiar with the story of Daniel, after taking Jerusalem, Nebuchadnezzar, the King of Babylon, told his chief eunuch that he should bring some of the children from the royal families of Israel "those with no blemish, handsome in appearance, skilled in all wisdom, cunning in knowledge and understanding of science" and they were to be brought to the palace. There they would be fed and nourished from the king's own meats and delicacies for three years so they might then stand and minister to the King. Daniel was one of the boys brought to the palace, but he requested from the prince of the eunuchs that he and three others not be made to defile themselves by eating the meat and delicacies the King had so generously provided them. The head eunuch was afraid that the king would have him beheaded for disobeying, but Daniel challenged him and said "test your servants for 10 days; and let them give us vegetables (pulse) to eat and water to drink." At the end of 10 days Daniel and his friends won every challenge (physical and mental) as well as looked much better than those who had been eating the king's meats and drinking the king's wine. After Daniel and the others had proven the superiority of their diet, the head eunuch let them continue eating like that for the next three years. When they finally came before King

Nebuchadnezzar, "he found none among all of them like Daniel, Hananiah, Mishael and Azariah, and in all matters of wisdom and understanding that the king inquired of them, he found them ten times better than all the magicians and astrologers in his whole realm."[1]

For the non-Christian reader and those with the typical western mind set, the next two sections with their scientific data and logic, combined with the fact that much of this diet is just common sense, will help you get beyond the initial stage. I know that once you've tried it for awhile, the odds are greatly increased that you'll never return to your old way of living. For the millions of people that don't really care about spiritual matters, don't worry, the proof is in the pudding. I guarantee you'll get benefits you never imagined by following this simple way of living even without the benefits in the wake-up section.

---

[1] King James Bible; Daniel 1; Verses 1-2; also Holy Bible George Lamsa's Translation Daniel 1; Verses 1-21

How It Works

One of the big problems with most diets is that they're just too complicated and rigid. They may be on solid ground medically and nutritionally, but if they're hard to live with, not taking into account how the person operates in real life, they are doomed to failure. That is why the percentage of people that gain most of their weight back in the first year is so staggering.

In marked contrast, "Jesus' DieT..." was created to be simple, flexible and to have few rules. In fact, it's a lifestyle much more than a diet and it's meant to last for a lifetime, not three months or a year. There's no weighing food, or counting calories, carbohydrates or proteins, and certainly no figuring out your numbers after finding out your body/fat ratio. There are no portions to be thought out either as this diet is based on common sense, allowing for human frailty. You can cheat and even go on the occasional binge vacation once you know the basic rules. Then following the break you can go back to phase one for a week or do a short fast afterwards. There are even plenty of desserts that are fair game for those people that don't find their sweet tooth has vanished entirely. In other words you can bend and break most all of the rules once you understand how to undo the damage and get back on track.

Most of us lead complicated enough lives without having food and hunger be a part of the problem. Your main concern becomes simply learning which are the life generating and life sustaining foods, the good carbs and good fats, and learning to supplement your enzymes, thereby helping the entire process along by chewing your food better. You'll find portions, percentages, and ratios all end up taking care of themselves because you simply won't be hungry!

The pillar of this entire way of living is to replace bad carbs with good carbs and bad fat with good fat while learning to eat some of the alternative sources of protein – that's it! Since no two people are alike, each person has to find where he is comfortable. The goal is to create your own version within the basic rules, a version that is flexible and adaptable to your tastes, habits and lifestyle while still allowing foods you love to eat. Just starting to ask the question of whether or not a food is life-enhancing, life-sustaining, life-debilitating or life-destroying will start the ball rolling.

Remember, the more food is processed the more fattening it is. You want sugar to be released gradually – this is crucial to understand. Once you understand the principle behind releasing insulin slowly into your blood stream you're home free.

Let's take a potato for instance. You'd think baked would probably be the best for your system. Wrong! It's actually the worst because it renders the starch easily accessible to your digestive system. Believe it or not, by adding a dollop of cheese or sour cream you've just made it better as the fat will slow down the process which lessens the amount of insulin your body needs to make. Best would be to mash or boil them and add butter or sour cream. The type of potato is also a factor as red skinned potatoes are higher in carbs than white skinned and sweet potatoes are the best of all.

Remember that all fruits and vegetables have a lower carb count when picked younger and try to buy produce that is grown close to home and as fresh as possible. Take an afternoon to locate all your local produce stands and go ask a few pertinent questions before settling on one. A little extra drive time to find a country stand will pay huge dividends over the long run.

All natural peanut butter is much better than the typical processed variety at your local super market, but use as little jelly as possible or look into one of the pure fruit jellies and jams that have been created lately. We can thank The Zone, South Beach and Atkins plans for motivating manufacturers to create numerous choices in the low carb arena. When it comes to your lingering sweet tooth I would take full advantage of their priming the market.

Want the occasional banana split, no problem. Just substitute berries for the banana and add walnuts and almonds. It may be loaded with sugar but the good fat will keep away the cravings afterwards. Most people make the mistake of using low-fat ice cream when you actually want the fat. In other words you can break the rules, but do it knowledgeably.

Here's a surprise to most people. Rice cakes are a no-no and white bread is worse than ice cream.[1] You want the fibers that aren't processed because they delay your stomach's effort to get to the sugar and starches. Fats and proteins also slow down the process, so a little olive oil on your bread is an improvement over eating bread by itself.

When it comes to fluids, water is best and you should try and drink two or three quarts daily. Beer is the worst because of the high glycemic index in maltose. Fruit juices are not as good as vegetable juices and should be consumed accordingly. We've been programmed to believe that apple or orange juice for breakfast is healthy when actually you might as well just eat six spoonfuls of sugar. You'll get a huge sugar rush and then crash almost as fast. This is a perfect example to show how it's really your eating that is making you hungry. Most of us have been doing it for so long that we are numb to the effects, but once you break your cravings and can get back in touch with your body signals, you'll see just what I mean.

When it comes to indulging in desserts, the chewing rule should be arduously practiced. It's amazing to find three to four bites, if chewed slowly and savored, is just as satisfying as cleaning your plate. If you have to occasionally eat the whole thing that's OK too, just make sure the sweetener used in preparing it was Stevia, fruit juice, or rice syrup and that the fat used in preparation was one of the good ones. As a general rule, pass up the desserts in public and stick to the ones prepared at home where you can know what you're eating. In the fruit department, they're all life sustaining and you really can't go wrong. Bananas, pineapple and mango all have high glycemic levels and are great to break fasts with. Blueberries,

---

[1] Arthur Agatston, M.D. "The South Beach Diet", 2003, St. Martins Press

blackberries, raspberries, strawberries, cherries, apples, plums,
pears, apricots, nectarines, pomegranates, grapes, coconuts,
melons, peaches, you can take your pick. The number of flavors
and combinations that are possible is practically endless.
Watermelon, cantaloupe and honeydew are great but are preferable
when eaten alone.

When you do breakfast, remember the word means break fast.
Whole fruits are an excellent way to start. Any natural grain cereals
such as kashi are good but unless you know the source of your
milk, switch to soymilk or rice dream (you'll understand why after
the next chapter). Slow cooked non-processed oatmeal is an option
that will give you a slow burning fuel and leave you feeling satisfied
as well. Any omelet with cheese, asparagus, spinach, soy sausages
can be eaten and you might try different spices and salsas for added
variety. Eat only eggs that come from free range chickens as the
typical store bought variety have much more cholesterol and toxins
in them. Whole grain waffles and pancakes are OK, but use brown
rice syrup, honey, or a sweet fruit topping. Fritattas with salsa are
OK – but always choose the whole grain products, remembering
white flour, white sugar and processed foods are your enemy. Also
remember anything cooked loses its enzymes, so have a basic
enzyme supplement available. The more you stick with living foods
the better.

Many people are beginning to at least suspect what it means to
have a healthy diet, but one thing everyone knows for sure is that
nothing is much fun when you don't feel well. Unfortunately very
few people have any idea how much better they could feel if they
chose to change their diet. It's the old adage "you don't miss what
you've never had."

There are many advances in nutrition and science available that
have shed new light on the importance of food combining and the
difference between good fat and bad fat and good carbohydrates
and bad carbohydrates. These advances clearly need to be understood if you truly want all the gusto life has to offer. Here are some
of the scientific explanations behind why "Jesus' DieT…" works
and why simplifying your way of eating is in your best interest.

Diet Plan: The Three Phases

"The natural healing force within us is the greatest force in getting well."

— Hippocrates, Father of Medicine

Since the dawn of man we have been genetically disposed to store fat as a survival technique for times of famine. Unfortunately, or fortunately depending on how you look at it, we no longer have famines in this country so we are never required to burn off the excess fat we have stored. Meanwhile, most of the changes in our preparation of foods have been changes for the worse. Baked goods, breads, snacks, and processed foods are all metabolized differently than the foods our forefathers ate. They all turn to sugar quickly which then spikes the insulin level. This in turn causes a chemical reaction in the body or brief surge of energy that has a resultant mandatory let down. It's the law, and just like the law of gravity it's going to happen whether you want it to or not. We then have to eat again to experience that same addictive surge and it starts the pattern all over again. This pattern we now know to be extremely unhealthy. I'll repeat it once again, *it's your eating habits that are making you think you're hungry.*

It's probably a good time to point out that much of what is passed off as food in our culture is not food at all. Food by its very definition is supposed to build, sustain, nourish, repair and replenish our bodies, while much of what is available at today's supermarkets does just the opposite. Many of today's choices have none of the above qualities; while they destroy the very living organism it is supposed to be helping. Here's Webster's definition:

FOOD   Function: noun

1 a : material consisting essentially of protein, carbohydrate, and
    fat used in the body of an organism to sustain growth, repair
    vital processes and to furnish energy; *also* : such food
    together with supplementary substances (as minerals,
    vitamins, and condiments) b : inorganic substances absorbed
    by plants in gaseous form or in water solution

2 : *nutriment in solid form*

3 : something that nourishes, sustains, or supplies; food for
   thought

Let's look further at the question of good carbs versus bad carbs.
Good carbs are those that release energy slow and steady into the
bloodstream like most vegetables, or oatmeal, while the bad carbs
are those that boost your insulin in a hurry such as orange juice,
fast food snacks and cereals covered in sugar. Once you decrease
the bad carbs, the insulin resistance starts to clear on its own and
the cravings stop. After awhile, the blood chemistry in the body will
go back to normal which will help all your bodily systems and
functions.

The number one principle to remember here is to build your diet
on the good carbs (fruits, vegetables, whole grains, nuts etc.) and
curtail the bad carbs, especially those highly processed foods that
have been stripped of all nutritional value through the manufactur-
ing process. This is very contrary to the Atkins Diet that keeps the
focus on protein, allowing limitless saturated fat found in red meat
and butter while banning most carbs. In the long run you're asking
for trouble, in fact, that's the problem. That way of eating almost
guarantees you *won't have a long run*. You're feeding mostly dead
foods into a system that thrives on live ones. Sure you might lose
some weight in the short term, but it's not nearly as safe *(or nearly
as quick)* as following nature's way of fasting and then rebuilding
your body with life-sustaining foods.

Since we live in the real world, and I know there will be some of
you that can't go cold turkey (no pun intended) on all meats, you
can start by weaning yourself gradually to just fish. Once you learn
some of the details on how most commercial meats come to be in
your local grocery, it will undoubtedly make the weaning process a
whole lot easier. Personally, the only meat I would let anywhere
close to my mouth anymore would be free-range chickens and
turkeys found at most health food markets, and even then I'd
double check to find out how the animals were raised. It's
important to understand that once meat is cooked, you kill off all
the enzymes and are inserting a dead food into a system that thrives
on live substances. I'm convinced that's what Jesus was referring to

when he told us repeatedly, "by eating the dead we turn our own bodies into tombs." You'll be amazed, by just banishing the dead and processed foods like meat, white flour, white sugar and white pasta, how fast your body starts to go back to its natural weight and get back in a rhythm of health like you were intended to experience.

Phase One – Break the Cravings

This phase lasts two weeks, and the goal here is to help you break any and all of your life long craving cycles. To accomplish this we're going to bend some of the rules to not only wean you off your old habits, but so you can lose between six and 10 pounds (typically off your mid section). In this phase we will eliminate the urges so the weight loss isn't from eating less food, but from eating less food that creates the old cravings. If you're already in pretty good internal shape you might choose to start with a short three to five day juice or water fast where people typically lose between two to three pounds a day.

Eat plenty of vegetables, (free range) eggs, yogurt, nuts, some fruits, soymilk, veggie burgers (without bread), humus, salsas, soy sausages and links that can taste surprisingly like meat. One admonition you can't cheat on, is to drink lots of water and carry it with you always. The occasional diet colas are OK for now, but you want to start getting used to lots of water as the colas can be quite addictive. In this first phase, while you're breaking the cravings, you can cheat on the eventual goal of two meals a day. In fact I recommend doing three meals a day with a couple snacks in between during this early stage. Think of it as breakfast, lunch and dinner with two picker-uppers in between. Don't worry, you'll still lose the weight. During this phase if you absolutely have to eat some meat, then stick to fish (salmon, tuna or mackerel).

Boredom is typically the main enemy here. So learn to take advantage of all recipes with herbs and spices, especially ones with intense flavors like horseradish, onions, garlic, hot peppers, cinnamon and nutmeg. Make big use of creative substitutions.

No fruit juices especially orange, no alcohol of any type, and by

all means, no white sugar, white flour, or pasta of any kind
including potatoes and rice. No starches of any kind. For oils stick
to mono and polyunsaturated fats like olive and peanut as these are
the good fats. Don't start your weekly one day fast till after we've
broken the cycle of cravings.

Phase Two: Fasting–
Nature's Cure For What Ails You

"I saw few die of hunger – Of eating, a hundred thousand" –
Benjamin Franklin

You'll stay on this phase till you reach your optimal weight but
now you have three choices how to get there. Rapidly, gradually or
somewhere in between. All three choices are quite safe if you
follow the rules as I'll explain. The speed you decide you want to
lose weight should really depend on your personality, your current
state of health, and knowing from your past history if you have the
will power it requires to stick with the prolonged method. In most
diets, this second phase is usually where people get discouraged
after a month or two, as the weight loss slows to one or two
pounds a week and for most of us five pounds a month when your
goal is to lose 40 pounds can feel like an eternity – believe me, I
know. Don't worry, nature has an amazing solution that every other
creature on the planet does naturally except for man. It's called
fasting and is tried and true as it has been around for thousands of
years.

Nothing can circumvent the fact that the quickest, surest, safest
way to lose weight is by following nature's own guidepost, while
the surest way of maintaining the proper weight is by refusing to
return to your old bad habits afterwards. There have been many
scientific studies by the medical community that bear this out. Here
are just some of the advantages of fasting for weight reduction.[1]

1. Safe rapid loss from the fast (two to three pounds a day is
    standard)

---

[1] Shelton, Herbert "Fasting Can Save Your Life," 1964, Natural Hygiene Press

2. Easier than the reducing diet as the nagging desire to eat leaves in three days
3. Weight loss occurs without flabbiness or sagging of skin.
4. Breathing becomes freer
5. Greater sense of movement
6. Enhanced energy
7. Problems with indigestion cease
8. Blood pressure is lowered and the load on the heart is eased dramatically

One of the reasons the disappointingly slow method of dieting is rarely successful is because the long drawn out process requires more self control over a longer period of time than most people are capable of. The typical outcome is that the person loses an initial few pounds and then returns to their old habits while regaining the lost weight, along with additional pounds as well.

The wonderful thing about fasting is how little willpower is required as you won't feel hunger at all once you're into your third or fourth day. In fact, just the opposite occurs once the gastric juices are no longer being constantly activated, and your taste buds quit tempting you. That in itself produces a comfort I never get when I diet. Best part, besides seeing two to three pounds drop off a day of course, is that there is very little weakness and the hunger cravings totally disappear at some point. During a water fast, it's not unusual to see a person lose 15-20 pounds in a week as it is the body itself which prescribes how much weight loss is proper. After that it slows down to about one pound a day.

Fasting really is the easier softer way to lose weight and regain one's health and yet few people have experienced its amazing results. One of the key reasons is that most people confuse fasting with starving. Folks, there is a huge difference.

> "To fast is to abstain from food while one possesses adequate reserves to nourish the vital tissues; to starve is to abstain from food after the reserves have become exhausted so that vital tissues are sacrificed."[2]

Don't worry, your body will warn you when it has nearly

---

[2] Ibid note 34, page 30

exhausted its reserves, because hunger returns with such an
intensity you can't miss it. During the fast proper though, there is
almost no desire for food at all. Many people find this
phenomenon to be a small miracle. The reason behind it is that the
human body has a built in pantry that is completely stored up for
those times of famine. Since modern man no longer experiences
famine, the storehouse keeps piling up more and more reserves,
better known as all that extra fat you're now trying to get rid of.
Here's what Herbert Shelton had to say:

> "There are sufficient stores of protein, fat, sugar, minerals, and
> vitamins stored in the fat of the body, as well as in the blood, the
> lymph, the bones, in the marrow of the bones, in the liver and
> other glands for all the nutriment we require for prolonged
> periods of fasting. It is significant that even in prolonged fasting
> (of 60-90 days) no beriberi, pellagra, rickets, scurvy or other
> "deficiency disease" ever develops. Thousand of observations of
> both man and animals have established the fact that when the
> organism goes without food, the tissues are called upon in the
> inverse order of their importance to the organism. Thus, fat is the
> first to go. The stored reserves are used up before any of the
> functioning tissue of the body are called upon to supply nutrients
> for the more vital tissues….the fasting organism exercises an
> ingenuity that seems almost superhuman."[3]

Granted, Herbert Shelton isn't the only authority on fasting and
his view might be considered controversial by some. But he did
study its effects on people for decades and there are countless
testimonials to its benefits, while there are but few to its detriments
by people that have actually fasted themselves. One of the biggest
problems today is that most people don't really know when they're
hungry. We use food to cover up psychological discomforts just as
the drunkard uses alcohol to drown his. Few communities or
individuals in the western world have ever experienced genuine
hunger as we have cultivated the habit of eating by the clock, often
to the point we will persist in eating even when it seems repugnant.

"Finish your plate."

"No dessert until you've eaten everything else on your plate."

---

[3] Ibid note 34 page 29

"The doctor told you to eat this."

"You have to eat to keep your strength up"

Often, what we really need is just the opposite to get our strength back and system flowing again. It is only ignorance and force of habit that allows us to keep passing on these false truisms to our children.

It's important to note that fasting is not merely refraining from eating for a required time. Whether the objective is to reduce weight, lower blood pressure, relieve accumulated wastes, rest a tired nervous system, or just to rejuvenate the individual – it involves rest, sun baths, bathing, peace, quiet, drinking plenty of good water and especially careful preparation for how the fast will be broken.

As to how long one should fast, there are varying views and much discussion. The two basic facts I found across the board concerning long fasts were: 1) that one would know it was time to break the fast when hunger returned again, and 2) you will know it's time to break the fast when your breath turned sweet.

Though this isn't always practical, as a rule of thumb it is rarely wise to set an arbitrary limit to the duration of the fast. No man is wise enough to predetermine the amount required for the individual. In reality the best course of action is to take it day by day guided by the developments in the body of the person fasting. There are numerous documented cases of people having gone 60-70 days and even longer with no ill effects, but in general most people will get the greatest benefit somewhere between 14 and 40 days. Almost anyone can fast from 3 to 7 days safely though I recommend anything over 10 days should be supervised by a professional.

Armed with these facts I figured I'd go at least 3 days for my first water fast, as I was extremely curious if it was true that I'd lose my hunger as all the books claimed. Not only was it true, but I felt so good I decided to go a bit longer while paying attention to my body's own signals. I lost 15 pounds the first week and found I still wasn't hungry, so I decided to keep going until I was. I kept a journal of that entire first experience which now reminds me it was nothing short of extraordinary. The longer I fasted the more

fascinated I became with the entire process and started researching
at length the various studies on the subject. I was amazed to
discover that my physical energy and mental clarity was off the
charts. Four to five hours sleep nightly was all my body required
and I saw more sunrises than I'd seen in the previous 30 years. My
typical day would begin around 5am and usually go past midnight.
The occasional times I felt my energy wane I would just take it easy
and read a book, take a water bath or a sun bath or even an
afternoon nap. Another phenomenon that occurred during the fast
had to do with parasites.

I had come across a good bit of data about how the typical
American has parasites growing throughout their systems, and how
autopsies have revealed people with literally hundreds of feet of
these things in them at their deaths. I didn't think much about it
until days 21-24 of my fast, during which I passed 60 one foot
sections myself. It seems I had starved them to death. They were
made of a black rubbery substance as big as my little finger with
polyps attached every few inches. I continued fasting till day 36
and then stopped (half out of boredom and half wanting to have
the proverbial 40 day fast to look forward to sometime in the
future). I can report that though my hunger still hadn't returned,
my breath had turned sweet as promised. Now let's get back to
fasting.

Jesus had something very definite to say on the subject when
asked how long one should fast: He tells the story of the prodigal
son being gone for seven years and says the Heavenly Father allows
you to pay your debt of seven years in seven days of fasting. At that
point a sick man who suffered horribly asked him:

> "…and if we have sinned for seven times seven years?" and Jesus
> answered him: "Even in that case the Heavenly Father forgives
> you all your debts in seven times seven days … each day that you
> continue to fast and to pray, God's angels blot out one year of
> your evil deeds from the book of your body and your spirit."

Ideally, longer fasts of two weeks or more should be supervised
by a professional or conducted at an institution in which fasting is
regularly carried out. This is especially important if it's your first
long one. For many people the first fast can be a most unusual

experience and they might experience periods of unfounded anxiety or uncertainty about what they're doing. Having a professional to guide them through those times is quite helpful. If that isn't possible and one chooses to do it at home, it should be in quiet, peaceful surroundings where the air and water are pure and uncontaminated, and the people around you are congenial. I strongly advise people on doing their homework and reading up on fasting at great length to have a better idea of what they're embarking upon. Arnold Ehret's, Herbert Shelton, Edmond Bordeaux Szekely, and Paul C Bragg as well as numerous others have written at great length of this wondrous practice that has healed and transformed so many lives.

Here are just a few of the comments that followers of Braggs live food and fasting program had to say on the subject.

"Bragg saved my life at age 15..." Jack LaLanne

"Paul Braggs work on fasting and water is one of the great contributions to Healing Wisdom in the world today." Gabriel Cousins, MD Conrad Hilton – founder of Hilton Hotels, J.C. Penny and Dr. Scholl's, the foot Magician, all gave Bragg and his fasting program credit for enhancing their lives. Other fasters you might have heard of include Steven Spielberg, Barbara Streisand, Christie Brinkley, Alec Baldwin, Donna Karan, Daryl Hannah, Clint Eastwood and Cloris Leachman who said: "Fasting is simply wonderful. I can do practically anything. It's a miracle cure. It cured my asthma."

Before my first fast I spent hours and hours on the computer researching and reading hundreds of testimonials of other people's experiences, and then equally as much time preparing for how I planned to break the fast as well.

Here are a few of the basic rules I discovered:

1. **Preparation** – It's important to understand the wisdom and rationale and rid your mind of all fear around this perfectly natural process. If you have any fear you haven't researched it or spoken to enough people that have done it.

2. **Rest** – Bear in mind "in order to expend on one side, nature must conserve on the other." What you don't expend in unneeded activity is available for use in elimination and

repair. I'm not talking about total passivity, but absence of
strain so the physical sense of peace becomes possible.

3. **Activity** – In reducing fasts, some moderate exercise is OK,
   but in any other type, needless expenditure of energy should
   be avoided. (I broke this rule religiously.)

4. **Warmth** – People fasting get cold easily and that inhibits
   elimination and causes a more rapid utilization of reserves.

5. **Water** – The normal demand for water should be met with
   the purest water available. A distilled or filtered water is best.
   There is nothing to be gained by drinking large quantities on
   the theory that it flushes out the system. True that it does
   make the kidneys work over time, but this does not increase
   the elimination of waste.

6. **Bathing** – A minimum of one bath a day and should cause
   the least expenditure of energy. Bath water should be
   lukewarm, as it requires considerable energy to resist both
   hot and cold.

7. **Sunbathing** – Sunlight is an essential nutrient factor in both
   plant and animal nutrition and is helpful while fasting. It is of
   far greater importance than most people realize. Preferably
   early morning sun while it is still cool or late afternoon when
   the temperature is comfortable.

8. **Purges** – Enemas, colonics, saline purges and such are
   recommended by some in the field and not so by others. Do
   your own homework and see how it feels to you. I personally
   found starting my fast off with a colonic and then doing a
   cleansing enema every other day felt right, but like I said,
   everyone seems to have a different opinion about this. Jesus
   left us a very clear roadmap on the subject 2000 years ago.

   "He who cleanses himself without, but within remains unclean,
   is like to tombs that outwards are painted fair, but are within, full
   of all manner of horrible uncleanesses and abominations. So I tell
   you truly, suffer the angel of water to baptise you also
   within…seek therefore a large trailing gourd, having a stalk (hose)
   the length of a man, take out its inwards (make the tube hollow as
   well as the gourd) and fill it with water from the river which the
   sun has warmed. Hang it upon the branch of a tree, and kneel

upon the ground before the angel of water, and suffer the end of the stalk of the trailing gourd to enter your hinder parts, that the water may flow through to your bowels...then let the water run out of your body, that it may carry away from within it all the unclean and evil-smelling things of Satan."

There's a wonderful story about Isaac Jennings, M.D. (1788-1874) who spent the first 20 years of his practice adhering to the drugging and bleeding out practices of his time. He gradually realized people weren't improving all that much and that many of them improved more when he didn't put them on drugs. He decided to change his methods and instead started giving them placebos he had created in both pill and liquid form. At the same time he would advise them on diet and proper rest and instructed them to use the placebo "medicine" with no food and only water for the first week. He warned them the medicine would not be effective if they didn't follow his directions. He usually continued their imposed fast for a few days after that first week was up. Diseases started vanishing and his fame began to spread. People thought his medicines were magic potions and he became the greatest healer of his day – all from fasting and change of diet.

More Phase Two

If the rapid method of weight loss (fasting) doesn't appeal to you, or if you'd rather prepare yourself more gradually before jumping in, you can start by doing the weekly one day fast to get a feel for it. Pick a day that affords you the most leisure like a Saturday or a Sunday and follow the other rules about fasting. Some people like to begin with one day water fasting followed by two days juice fasting and then a pause. Then two days water and three days juice etc., but like most people, since I find it's the first two to three days that are the toughest days anyway, this method doesn't appeal to me. I want to get over the hump and get on to the good stuff and watch the weight literally melt away. You might want to prepare by switching to a plant based diet for at least two weeks like we did in phase one before beginning. Once you've started to clean out your body, and learned about the art and science of fasting, you can always begin a longer fast later.

In this slower version of phase two, you definitely want to start adding back the fruits, especially the berries, apples and grapefruits as well as adding back some of your indulgences such as a good hearty dark bread, potatoes (sweet is best), and even chocolate. Thanks to Atkins, there are some amazing low carb bars in your local health food store that will give a Nestle's Crunch Bar a run for their money. Keep in mind, however, most of your old indulgences are dead foods with no living properties, so start thinking in terms of living foods. This would also be a great time to start exploring the world of sprouts. The nutritional value you get by just adding a pile to your daily salad can't be beat. It takes a little effort at first, but they're incredibly inexpensive and easy to do at home with just a few wide mouth jars, some cheese cloth and rubber-bands.

Eventually you'll want to change over to natural sweeteners such as Stevia or brown rice syrup which allows you to make a wide variety of desserts. Again, do the sweets only in moderation so your sweet tooth isn't feeling deprived. You have to use some discipline and pick and choose the indulgences you allow yourself. You can still enjoy them, but the idea is to learn to enjoy them differently so they no longer control your life.

It might be helpful to think of your body as your home where you're going to hopefully be living for a long time, and like any home, it needs rebuilding and repairing as it gets older. Now think of the vitamins, minerals, proteins, carbs and fats as the raw materials waiting to be put to use for those repair jobs that come up on occasion. Even though there may be an ample supply of raw building materials lying around, nothing can happen until the construction workers show up. These construction workers are better known to you as enzymes and they are truly that important. They literally run the show and yet, most of us are seriously deficient in them. We have government guidelines on vitamins and minerals, even protein, fats and carbohydrates, but none on enzymes. Why? Because those in power in our health industry say the body can make its own, unlike vitamins and minerals. In an ideal world they are right, but not in the world we live today, and though that attitude will undoubtedly change in the 21st century, in the meantime, millions of people are paying the price for that lack of public awareness.

It's true our body does make enzymes, but unfortunately they have to rob Peter to pay Paul. While they should be repairing cells, tissues, organs and entire body systems, they are busy trying to digest all the garbage of the average modern diet. That's not an exaggeration. You walk down the aisle of any grocery store and almost all you see is dead food. Food with absolutely zero enzymes. Practically everything you eat from a box, a bag, a bottle or a can is dead food. As soon as you eat it your body has to supply enzymes to make it usable in the body. Remember, the real point of eating is to feed nutrition into the body so it can build and repair all the various systems and trillions of cells at work, not just for the purpose of getting full. Unfortunately, most of what we eat these days does the direct opposite; it destroys and kills. Because of this, much of the vitamin and mineral supplementation we may get is wasted because there is an inadequate supply of enzymes (workers) to put them to use.

Enzymes must be removed from our food supply in order for food products to achieve extended shelf life. Chemists began figuring out just how to do that in the early part of the 20th century. They described enzymes back then as "the dreaded contaminant enzymes found in food."[1] One of the new areas of advancement (if you can call it that) is in growing hybrid foods such as tomatoes that will have a reduced amount of natural enzymes, which of course allows for greater shelf life. It's great for the grocer, but it will put even more of a strain on the body of the typical consumer who is getting very little enzymes elsewhere. Besides that, you'll discover that though those tomatoes look great, they have almost no taste. I imagine the growers of this "Frankenfood" are counting on people that have never tasted the real thing, and banking on the adage "you won't miss what you never had."

Right now, more than a billion dollars is being spent annually on drugs that relieve symptoms for people with indigestion; heartburn, bloating, excess acid and constipation. They do nothing to improve

---

[1] Loomis, Howard, "Enzymes –The Key To Health—Volume 1"

people's ability to digest food on their own and yet there's a "little
known secret" that could make a huge difference. "Each raw
uncooked fruit, vegetable or meat contains enzymes that will digest
the food in which they are contained."[2] The problem is that all the
enzymes are destroyed during cooking, canning, and food processing. Any temperature over 118 degrees will destroy that which
your body needs the most. What happens is our body has to
borrow enzymes from other tissues and organs, especially our
immune system, to complete digestion and the vicious cycle continues.
Another problem is the way most people are eating constantly, rarely
giving any breaks or (fasts) for the body to repair itself.

Most people that are overweight have low supplies of the enzyme
lipase in their bodies which is the enzyme which digests fat. Since
undigested fat is easily stored in your body, you definitely want to
get a good all around enzyme supplement going. For faster weight
loss you can even sprinkle it on your food at mealtimes. This not
only helps the digestive process, but also frees up your natural
enzymes for other jobs. One of the good things about taking
enzymes is that unlike vitamins or even proteins that aren't used up
and are eliminated, enzymes are never wasted but keep getting
added to the enzyme pool of your body. Plant enzymes by the way
are much preferable to animal enzymes. Go to Yahoo search engine
and type in enzyme and do some research. There are some charts
you can find that show which companies give you the most bang
for your buck and you can rest assured there is a huge difference.
The Health Nuts Ultimate Enzyme brand I've found to be a good
choice these days.

Now that we're in phase two it's important that we take an
entirely new approach to the way we look at foods and how we
categorize them. The old way obviously isn't working for a
majority of the people on the planet as the amount of cancers,
heart attacks, all forms of disease and obesity is on the rise.
Diseased bodies have become a way of life and the reality is, it just
doesn't have to be that way.

Edmund Bordeaux Szekely, founder of the Golden Door Health

---

[2] Ibid

Spa and author of "The Essene Gospel of Peace" taught us a much more user friendly way of looking at foods over fifty years ago. Instead of breaking our foods down into the basic categories of carbohydrates, proteins and fats, he believed it would be wiser to look at them as **life generating** ("biogenic"), **life sustaining** ("bioactive"), **life debilitating** ("biostatic"), and **life destroying** ("bioacidic").[3]

Life generating is the best of all possible food choices as it goes into your body while still alive with all the nutrients intact. Seeds, sprouts, fresh cut greens, whole grains, nuts and legumes would fit into this category.

Life sustaining includes all the fruits and vegetables, and raw unpolluted, non-pasteurized, unprocessed milks of the animals. These two categories (**life generating** and **life sustaining**) both accelerate cell renewal, cell respiration and strengthen the oxygen transport throughout the body while destroying any potentially harmful substances that may enter your body in this heavily chemicalized and polluted planet of ours. These foods are so easy on the system that they free up most of our enzymes to work on all our other areas of concern. This is important because they aren't free to do that in most people. At the very minimum, a healthy diet needs to be made using 75% of these two. Another reason to consume much of these foods (besides it being common sense to want the most nourishing food there is), is so they can then over-come the effects of the other 2 categories which actually slow down and often destroy the very processes of life they are supposed to be supporting. Amazingly, these other two categories are what most people subsist on.

This next category **life debilitating**, or "biostatic" as Szekely coined it, is basically the all American diet, and you can pretty much consider anything that is canned, packaged, frozen, bagged and preserved at your local market to fit into this category. All these foods slow down the life processes and accelerate the process of aging. *Period!* This would include most cooked foods, and any foods that aren't fresh. Meat, most eggs and most modern day

---

[3] Edmund Bordeaux Szekely "The Essene Way—Biogenic Living" published by Intnl Biogenic Society

dairy products slow down the life sustaining processes
tremendously. Modern meat is the biggest culprit of all. It takes
tremendous energy away from the other processes as your body has
to deal with digesting and then eliminating it while it could be
doing so many other worthwhile activities. Activities such as
healing your eyes, ears, organs, limbs and literally every other part
of your anatomy.

That by the way, is exactly what your body was created to do in
the first place. Only man in his modern day folly thinks he can
figure out a better system than what God started us out with in the
first place. Don't get me wrong. I'm all for some of the marvels of
modern day medicine when the need calls, but people would be
amazed to see what the body can do on its own if given half a
chance. Unfortunately, only a fraction of mankind even has a clue
to the miracle that is within each and every one of us already just
waiting to be called upon to go to work. Instead, we hear "how
does chicken McNuggets sound for dinner?"

The last category is called **life destroying** or (bioacidic) and these
should be avoided totally. These foods all contain harmful
substances such as additives, chemicals, adulterants, preservatives
and have been refined and processed which kills most, if not all of
their nutrient value as well.

Just learning to look at foods in this new/old way can make a
remarkable difference in your life. In fact, that one change in
consciousness alone could reap tremendous results if taken to
heart. Unfortunately, our modern day basic categories of protein,
carbohydrates, fats and starches denotes merely the chemical
composition of foods rather than the much more practical user-
friendly categories of life generating, life sustaining, life debilitating
or life destroying.

Phase Three - for life:

No longer a diet at all, but a way of living that you will come to
love once you've broken the cravings and lost the urges that were
chemically induced before. By now you will have lost the weight
while hopefully becoming more knowledgeable about the
importance of fasting, enzymes, and live foods, and have created a

routine that works for you. The energy and clarity that will accompany this stage is astounding to everyone that tries it. Typical comments are:

"I never knew I could feel this good." Or "Why did I wait so long to learn about this?" "It seems to be affecting every area of my life. All those years overweight when it really is simple once you know how."

Once you're at this stage, it's rare when someone goes back. Even if you break it with the occasional or routine binge, you can go back to phase one and be back where you want in no time. You will actually alter your blood chemistry to the long term benefit of your cardiovascular system, and you will dramatically increase the odds at not only living a long life, but having much better health and vitality as you age. Speaking of which… *ANYBODY BESIDES ME INTERESTED IN HAVING A LONG LIFE WHERE THE YEARS 75-100 MIGHT BE CONSIDERED SOME OF YOUR BEST?*

Longevity

No, I haven't lost my mind. This is the well documented outcome of living by the tenets of this kind of diet. Calcas from Peru died in 1761 at the age of 140. Pari from Chile, whom Alexander Hunboldt tells us about after having spent time with him at the age of 143. We know about Louis Truxo who died in 1780 at the age of 175. Jose Moreira and Sabina of Lemos, both of Brazil lived to be 115 and died in 1869 and 1872, respectively. How about Thomas Carn, who survived 12 kings of England having been born in London in 1588 and living till the ripe age of 207 before dying in 1795? There's the Countess Desmond Catherine who lived to be 145 and kept her beauty till her very last years. You can read the biography of Jenkins who was born in Yorkshire in 1500 and died at Bolton in 1670. Both his sons by the way lived to be over a hundred as well. How about Charlotte Dessen of Temeesvar, the wife of Jean Rovin. They lived to be 164 and 172 respectively and were married 147 years. (Keep in mind most of these people were living in a time when the average life expectancy was less than 50 years of age.) Here are the words of Luigi

Cornaro, a Venetian nobleman who changed his diet at the age of
40 after being told he didn't have long to live as he was quite ill
having "lived a careless and dissipated life like the majority of
young men in his day."[1] He changed his diet and learned about
fasting and lived to be 102. Here are his words to consider:

"Some sensual unthinking persons affirm, that a long life is no
great blessing, and that the state of man who has passed his
seventy-fifth year, cannot really be called life; but this is wrong, as I
shall fully prove; and it is my sincere wish, that all men would
endeavor to attain my age, that they might enjoy *that period of life
which of all others is most desirable.* I will therefore give an account
of my recreations, and the relish which I find at this stage of my
life. There are many who can give testimony as to the happiness of
my life. In the first place, they see with astonishment the good state
of my health and spirits; how I mount my horse without assistance,
how I not only ascend a flight of stairs, but can climb a hill with
greatest ease. Then how gay and good-humored I am; my mind
ever undisturbed, in fact joy and peace having fixed their abode in
my breast. I pass my hours in great delight and pleasure, in
converse with men of good sense and intellectual culture; then
when I cannot enjoy their company, I betake myself to the reading
of some good book. When I have read as much as I like, I write,
endeavoring in this, as in other things, to be of service to
others….my senses thank God, are perfect, particularly my palate,
which now relishes better the simple fare I have, than it formerly
did the most delicate dishes, when I led an irregular life. I can sleep
everywhere soundly and quietly and my dreams are pleasant and
delightful…..the memory tenacious, the body lively and strong, the
movements regular and easy; *and the soul, feeling so little of her
earthly burden, experiences much of her natural liberty.* The man
thus enjoys a pleasing and agreeable harmony, there being nothing
in his system to disturb; for his blood is pure, and runs freely
through his veins, and the heat of his body is mild and temperate."[2]

The cultures with the very longest life spans are the Vilcambas
who reside in the Andes of Ecuador, the Abkhasians who live on

---

[1] Szekely, E.B. "The Essene Science of Fasting"
[2] Ibid

the Black Sea in the USSR, and the Hunzas who live in the Himalayas of Northern Pakistan. Researchers have found a "striking similarity" in the diet of these three groups, scattered though they are in different parts of the world. All three are either vegetarian or close to it.[3]

Studies closer to home are the numerous ones on the of mortality rates for Seventh Day Adventists (a conservative Christian group which provides both dietary and lifestyle advice to its members.) They are prohibited completely from using alcohol, tobacco and pork and strongly discouraged from using any meat, fish, eggs and caffeine type beverages. Because the latter is only discouraged and not prohibited, there is a wide range of consumption of these products. Also since many people don't come to the church till adulthood, many of these Adventists have been eating a diet high in animal products most of their lives. There have been multiple scientific studies done on this group and this is on average what they have found:

1. "As a whole male Adventists live an average of 8.9 years longer than the rest of non-smoking America while the women live an average of 7.5 years longer. The one's who live the longest are those that have been vegetarians the longest and for those who have been vegetarians over half their lives, the difference jumps to 13 years more added to their life span as opposed to non-smoking Americans."[4] 2. Egg and meat consumption is strongly associated with all causes of mortality. Dairy and milk consumption is the same with prostrate cancer. In nearly all the studies the earlier one switched to a vegetarian diet the lower the risk of coronary heart disease. 3. The more leafy green vegetables consumed the longer the life span. This confirmed once again the importance of raw natural plant foods and the loss of important qualities with cooking out the nutrients.[5]

---

[3] John Robbins, "Diet for A New America" pg 154
[4] Ruckner, C., Hoffman J. "The Seventh Day Adventist Diet," Snowden DA, Animal Product consumption and mortality in Seventh Day Adventists "American Journal of Clinical Nutrition" 1988;48: 739-748, Kahn HA, Philip RL 21 year followup on 27,530 adult Seventh Day Adventists on mortality rates "American Journal of Epidemiology" 1984;119:775-787
[5] Furhman, Joel, MD "Fasting and Eating for Health" pgs 74, 75

Now About Protein – Myth or Reality?

The most frequently asked question about the vegetarian diet is about getting enough protein. First it should be pointed out as human animals we are not biologically built for a high protein diet. There is no question that metabolically there is scant difference between humans and the great apes that are overwhelmingly vegetarian, even though with their great strength, speed and agility they could easily find an abundance of animals they could kill for food. Just like these great apes, we were not built to function optimally on diets high in fat and protein. Hence, western man is plagued by cancer, heart attacks and all manners of auto-immune diseases.

This great misunderstanding actually began almost 80 years ago when two scientists published a study showing how rats, fed a high animal protein diet, grew faster than those who grew up on plant protein diet. We now know that rats and humans have very different protein requirements and that humans can easily get all their protein needs met from plant sources. We also now know that rats that grow and mature the quickest, also die the earliest. Did you know the vast majority of chickens consumed in America are now raised and brought to your table within seven weeks, whereas in the past, a natural healthy environment would have required 21 weeks? How do you think the factory meat industry accomplishes this seeming miracle-growth as it is standard in cows and pigs also? Chemicals and hormones that's how! That's what we are ingesting into our bodies that are designed to be fed with living foods.

Here's what Pritikin had to say:

"Vegetarians always ask about getting enough protein. But I don't know any nutrition expert that can plan a diet of natural foods resulting in protein deficiency…you only need 6% of total calories in protein and it's practically impossible to get below 9% in ordinary diets."[1]

A team of Harvard researchers investigating the effects of a strictly plant food diet found:

"It is difficult to obtain a mixed vegetable diet which will

[1] Pritikin N. quoted in Vegetarian Times, issue 43, pg. 21

produce an appreciable loss of body protein without resorting to high levels of sugars, jams and jellies and other essentially protein-free foods."[2]

Body builder Arnold Schwarzenegger has this to say on the subject:

> "Kids nowadays...tend to go overboard when they discover body building and eat diets consisting of 50-70% of protein – something I believe to be totally unnecessary...In my formula for basic good eating: eat about one gram of protein for every 2 pounds of body weight."[3]

To meet Arnold's quota, you'd do fine without meat, poultry or eggs and in fact if you ate only broccoli you'd get 4 times his suggested requirement.

Here's what the National Academy of Science says in their Recommended Dietary Allowances:

> "There is little evidence that muscular activity increases the need for protein."

Here's a very short list of world champion vegetarian athletes doing everything from karate, figure skating, tennis, bodybuilding, ski jumping, wrestling, boxing, football, weight lifting, triathlons, cycling, weight lifting, power-lifting, marathon running, swimming, gymnastics and, of course, winning the Mr. Universe contest:

Ridgely Adele – won 8 national championships in karate
Surya Bonaly – Olympic Figure Skating champion
Peter Burwash – won the Davis Cup in tennis
Andreas Cahling – champion body builder and gold medallist in
    ski jump
Chris Campbell – Olympic wrestling champion
Nicky Cole – first woman to walk to the North Pole
Ruth Heidrich – 6 time Ironwoman; USA track and field Masters
    champion
Keith Holmes – world champion middle weight boxer
Desmond Howard – Heisman trophy winner in football
Peter Hussing – European super heavy weight boxing champion
Debbie Lawerence – world record holder, women's 5k racewalk

---

[2] Hegsted, D. "The Vegetarian Diet" Journal of the American Dietetic Association 62-63, 1975
[3] Schwartzenegger, A., "Arnolds Body Building For Men", Simon and Schuster, 1981

Sixto Linares – world record holder, 24-hour triathlon
Cheryl Marek/Estelle Gray – world record holders, cross country
   tandem cycling
Ingra Manecki – world champion discus thrower
Bill Manetti – power lifting champion
Ben Mathews – U.S. Masters marathon champion
Dan Millman – world champion gymnast
Martina Navatilova – Tennis champion – not sure the number of
   Wimbledon titles
Paavo Nurmi – long distance runner, 9 Olympic medals and 20
   world records
Bill Pearl – 4 time Mr. Universe
Bill Pickering – world record holding swimmer
Stan Price – world weight lifting record holder, bench press
Murray Rose – won many swimming Olympic gold records and
   has world records
Dave Scott – 6 time winner of the Ironman triathlon
Art Still – Football MVP/Hall of Fame, Defense end, Buffalo Bills/
   Kansas City
Jane Welzel – U.S. National marathon champion[4]

[4] Robbins John, "The Diet Revolution"

The Modern American Diet Equals 'Slow Suicide'
(Having a Healthy Fear of Obesity, Infirmity and Corporate Greed)

This next chapter is for those of you sitting on the proverbial fence; those who still aren't sure whether it's worth the effort to make such a major change in your lifestyle and could use a bit more convincing in the scientific arena. Though you know you need to do something, neither the admonitions of Jesus, or the track record of Szekely's 123,000 patients has convinced you this living-foods based plan is for you, or you don't think you have the will power to stop your bad eating habits. Habits can be hard to break no doubt about it, especially ones that are as comfortable as our food addictions can be. As uncomfortable as it might be to admit it, the bacon and eggs, steaks, white flour, ice cream, sugar and salt snacks have been your best friends for a long time; always there when you needed them.

One thing that helps is to remember that instead of losing a friend you're making new ones, and like any new relationship it's going to take a little time to build up trust. I've found that once someone starts to look and feel dramatically better so quickly, the old habits begin to lose their hold on you, and for many people they will eventually leave altogether. Between my personal understanding of addictive behavior and my desire to keep this book succinct, I decided rather than fill up this last section with recipes, it was more important to have a section for newcomers in the early stages when the going can get tough.

As to good recipes, there's a myriad of mouth watering vegetarian recipes available at any health food store but for starters, go to the internet and type in "God's banquet table." Whether its nuts, fruits, salads, juices, making your own healthy butter, to preparing party snacks that look and taste inviting, it's all there. I printed out 60 pages of amazing recipes for everything you can imagine and have been thrilled with the results. For those of you with a life long sweet tooth, I highly recommend getting a dehydrator. With all the dried pears, pineapples and cherries you

can eat, as well as yogurt based chewy fruit rolls and peanut butter
chews that can be made and stored easily, I promise you won't feel
deprived.

Hard Data For The Lingering Skeptics

As a student of life as well as a motivational speaker, I've found
there are two great motivators in life and they both work; love and
fear. Up until now I've mainly addressed those people who are
moved to action through the power of love. Using the admonitions
of Jesus I've been dangling the carrot of safe and rapid weight loss
while gently prodding you with common sense, reason and logic
behind this way of life, while pointing out you're going to feel so
much healthier as well. I've also been touting more energy, clarity,
peace of mind and the marked improvement in your spiritual
connection if you're so inclined. Love is certainly my preferred tool
of motivation, but I would be derelict in my duty if I didn't offer
some hard data to those people that require fear to finally be
inspired into determined action.

I have no doubt these next few chapters will especially appeal to
those of you who only quit smoking once the proof was so
overwhelming and the stigma so great that you couldn't ignore it
any longer. If you fit into that category, then here's your wake up
call!

Let' start with the most obvious problem, obesity, and hence by
association, the 'Great American Food Machine' that is responsible.
It stands to reason that our bodies require food to become obese.
Not necessarily lots of food, just the wrong ones over a period of
time. Obesity in general, and the meat and dairy industries in
particular, have now replaced the tobacco industry as having the
dubious distinction of being able to say "we're number one" – the
number one killer in our society. Don't be surprised if soon you'll
start to see warnings put directly on the meat, dairy and poultry
packaging in our country as the evidence is becoming
overwhelming as to the health risks they represent.

'The Great American Food Machine' knows that it's coming and
are already trying to placate the public by making announcements

on the front pages of our newspapers. I guarantee the food giants
are going to start bombarding us with *NEW* and *IMPROVED*
advertising now that they've taken the first steps towards cleaning
up their act. Front page news on USA TODAY on July 1, 2003 –
"Under Fire, Food Giants Switch to Healthier Fare." They'd like to
make you think they've had a change of heart (and policy) because
'somebody at McDonald's loves you.' *Don't buy it – and I mean
that literally.* A closing comment in that same article from the
world's No.1 food giant, Nestle, about the proposed changes was
very telling. As spokesman Francois-Xavier Perroud put it, (Nestle)
has "no intention of going that route (the healthier one) – (it) might
not make sense in all markets."[1] *Doesn't make sense to give people
healthier food? Huh? Am I missing something?* Oh, sorry, I forgot
it's not about nutrition and health it's about making the most
money. *How naive of me.* And that's from the largest distributor of
food stuff in the world.

The reality is their real motivation is fear as stock analysts are
giving food stocks the ax, lawmakers are threatening a 'fat tax,' and
all the lawsuits looming make it appear as if they are about to
become the next 'Big Tobacco' for trial lawyers. What they've
proposed to do so far is like offering you a different seat on the
Titanic, or putting a Band-Aid on your knee when you really need
triple by-pass surgery. It's certainly better than nothing, but not
much. Instead of ham and cheese in Kraft's 'Lunchable' meal kits
we'll now see chicken and cheese and white flour pita bread.
Instead of re-working their entire menu knowing that meat and
dairy products are slowly killing people while processed food has
taken away all the nutrition value, they decide to cut back the
calories by 5-10%.[2] Instead of announcing they'll be switching to
Stevia or Barley Malt or even rice syrup for a sweetener and
organic whole wheat flour while eliminating all white flour and
white sugar from the snacks they push, they decide to dump a little
less sugar and make the packages smaller. It's way too little too late
and the next 30 pages are dedicated to showing you why.

[1] Horovitz, Bruce, USA Today, July 1, 2003, Front page money section
[2] Ibid, Front page article, page 2

"Just The Facts Ma'am, Just The Facts"

Most people already know that sugar does nothing good for you so I'm not going to spend a lot of time on that subject other than showing you some easy alternatives for that sweet tooth. More importantly, people need to realize that science and medicine have laboriously, systematically and emphatically debunked the myths around the *supposed* health benefits of two of our major food groups, meat and dairy. If the food giants want to try and push their products because they taste good, that's certainly truth in advertising and they're entitled. But to keep promoting that our bodies need them, when the evidence to the contrary is so overwhelming, is just plain out of integrity. In fact, let's call a spade a spade, it's a flat out lie! Modern science and medicine have irrefutably proven just the opposite. *Science has also proven beyond a shadow of a doubt that the few benefits these two food groups offer (such as protein and calcium), are easily replaced with other foods that don't have any of the attending dire consequences of meat and dairy.* When compared to the downside they have on our bodies, our health, and even the planet, the benefits from eating these two food groups are actually quite negligible.

The reality is that the profiteers of the 'Great American Food Machine' don't want consumers to know the truth about their industry. The burgeoning obesity problem is just the tip of the iceberg. Just below the surface there's the horrifying living conditions of the animals whose flesh, eggs and milk end up in your body. *To the profiteers, the connection between that and our cancer-ridden society definitely must not be made.* They also don't want you to know the huge environmental price we're paying and the enormous impact their industries are having on not just our country, but much of the world. Add to that, the gargantuan financial drain the government subsidies are costing you the taxpayer in the way of water and electricity and you'll see the reason they'd prefer you not know how much that hamburger is really costing. They're afraid if you did, the public outcry could very well shatter the foundation of their golden goose.

At this point the elite few making all the profit aren't too terribly worried as Americans have notoriously short memories and with a few changes they figure they can be back to business as usual in no time (with 5-10% less calories of course). What follows is just a small sampling of the facts the meat, poultry and dairy industries would prefer the public didn't know.

For those of you wanting the detailed, all encompassing picture, I highly recommend getting a copy of John Robbins bestsellers, *Diet For A New America* and *Food Revolution*. The author was heir apparent to the Baskin-Robbins dairy conglomerate when he walked away in order to stay in integrity. With his inside connections, he knew what was happening in the dairy and meat industries and couldn't abide with what they were saying and doing in their pursuit of the almighty dollar. I had the privilege of introducing John to Paul and Linda McCartney after his book first came out in the late 80's. Paul and Linda had embraced a vegetarian diet and were very involved in helping prevent cruelty to animals so introducing them to each other seemed like a good way for me to be of service. Little did I know that 14 years later I would become passionate about the same subject, only inspired from another direction.

Like John Robbins said:

"It's not the killing of the animals that is the chief issue here, but rather the unspeakable quality of the lives they are forced to live."

I'm sure that opinions will vary as to what are the chief issues, but regardless of how you feel about killing animals, the very least we should do for ourselves and our families is make sure the meat, dairy and eggs we do consume aren't from one of the animal factories. As you'll soon see in glaring statistics, greed and not health is the primary concern of the vast majority of the 'Great American Food Machine.' It doesn't matter that their products are helping us commit slow suicide, for them, that's just the price of doing business.

Robbins continues: "...thousands of impeccably conducted modern research studies now reveal that the traditional assumptions regarding our need for meats, dairy products and eggs have been in error. In fact it is an excess in these very foods which had once been the foundation of good eating habits, that is responsible for the epidemics of heart disease, cancer, osteoporosis and many other diseases of our time."[3]

This was written sixteen years ago. We now know we need to add obesity to that list. To that end, let's start with some of the propaganda we are bombarded with by the dairy industry which Robbins appropriately labeled *"Got BS?"*[4]

How Now Brown Cow?

I found it encouraging that when the dairy industry presented a series of ads with celebrities like Mark Spitz and Vida Blue proclaiming "Everybody Needs Milk," the FTC took legal steps towards prosecuting them, calling the advertisements, "False, misleading and deceptive." The milk industry quickly changed it to: "Milk has something for everybody." Said Kevin McGrady, a medical researcher, "Milk has something for everybody all right – higher blood cholesterol and increased risk of heart disease and strokes."[5]

You probably remember a lot of advertisements with milk mustaches worn by celebrities like Whoopi Goldberg, film producer Spike Lee, model Tyra Banks, basketball's Patrick Ewing and Dennis Rodman, and tennis's Venus and Serena Williams all promoting milk to lower the chances of osteoporosis in African Americans. I'm sure they believed they are doing a public service, but the FDA tells us otherwise. In fact, they say just the opposite is true, that there is no evidence at all that increased calcium from milk will help this malady.[6]

How about the ad that says milk is "Nature's perfect food?" The reality is there are now numerous well known doctors from Benjamin Spock, MD., to the Physician in Chief at John Hopkins Children's Center that have publicly and emphatically

[3] Robbins, J. "Diet For a New America," intro xv
[4] Ronnins, J. "Food Revolution"
[5] Ibid.
[6] Physicians Committee for Responsible medicine, "The Milk Mustache ads Are All Wet," Good Medicine, Spring 1999
[7] Davis Brenda, "The Response to the Dairy Farmers Rebuttal to Becoming Vegetarian", Fall 1996, Dairy Bureau of Canada

recommended against consuming dairy products at all.[7] Sure it's the perfect food, "perfect for a 200 pound calf!"

How about the ads telling us that 'diary products build stronger bones' in the elderly? In 1994 *The American Journal of Epidemiology* found otherwise. Elderly folks with the highest dairy consumption had double the risk of hip fracture compared to those with the lowest consumption.[8] The National Dairy Council then funded a study in which post menopausal women drank 3 additional glasses of skim milk per day. Trust me, the Dairy Council was not too thrilled with the findings that were published in the *American Journal of Clinical Nutrition*. They reported that the study showed the women who drank the additional milk actually lost more calcium from their bones than the control group of women who didn't.[9] Hmmm, what a surprise that must have been to the Dairy Council to find egg on their face instead of their preferred mustache!

Actually the calcium losing effect of animal protein had become well known in scientific circles years earlier after they'd done a survey in 33 countries and found "an absolutely phenomenal correlation" between the ration of plant and animal foods. The more plant foods the stronger the bones and fewer fractures. The more animal foods the weaker the bones and the more fractures they experience."[10]

Bet you didn't know milk products are priced by federal law according to a price structure that provides the dairymen more profit on higher fat products? The Dairy Council has such a grip over our schools that we have all been programmed to believe the extolling virtues of milk when nothing could be further from the truth. The lengths to which the 'saturated fat industries' are willing to go to defend their profits is quite amazing. In 1984 the US Government finally announced the results of the broadest, most expensive research in medical history. After ten year's of systematic research and more than 150 million dollars later, the director of the project, Basil Rifkind concluded:

[8] Cummings, R.G. "Case Controlled Study of Hip Fractures in Elderly" American Journal of Epidemiology, 1994
[9] Robbins, John
[10] US. News and World Report, Oct, 2000, Anthony Sebastian in article by Douglas Fox

"...strongly indicates that the more you lower cholesterol and fat in your diet, the more you reduce your risk of heart disease."[11]

My problem isn't that the dairy industry wants to sell us their product, hell, that's the American way! My problem is that their ads are deceptive, often untrue, and that they trick people intentionally into believing dairy products are necessary for a healthy diet. Implying your bones will break just isn't true as most Asian countries will attest. If the dairy industry wants to promote ice cream for the sheer hedonistic pleasure of the experience, no problem! Go ahead sell your products because they taste good on a hot day, but to imply untruths as they do in their advertising is a crime in my book.

Consider this one fact alone: Do you know why you see all the dairy propaganda in advertisements, but not on the milk cartons themselves? Because the FDA (Federal Drug Administration) won't allow false advertising! The FTC (Federal Trade Commission) on the other hand is much more lax about statements not backed up by facts.

The Cow Jumped Over The What? (Mad Cows R Us)

Now let's take a brief look at the beef industry. In 1985 the Beef Council had the dubious distinction of being a *repeat* winner of the "Harlan Page Hubbard Memorial Award" for the years most deceptive and misleading advertising. At this point, annual medical costs in the United States *directly attributable to meat consumption* are between 60-120 billion dollars.[12] This was the conservative estimate of Dr. Colin Campbell of Cornell University who headed the China Health Project, a joint Sino-American undertaking looking at the increased obesity and cancer rates in that country since they introduced an American style diet in 1978. Moreover, these changes occurred at a level of meat consumption only a fraction of the American intake.

Let's look at how the beef industry responded to these kinds of

---

[11] Robbins, J. "Diet For A new America"
[12] Halwell, Brian, "United States Leads World Meat Stampede" Worldwatch Issues Paper, July 2, 1998

findings that are becoming so numerous? National Cattlemen's website 2001:

"It's a myth that the risk of death from heart disease can be greatly reduced if a person avoids eating a meat centered diet." [13]

Unfortunately, the heart attack has become so much a part of American life that we just take it for granted. Consider what one well known publication wrote:

"A vegetarian diet can prevent 97% (ninety-seven) of our coronary occlusions."

I'm sure you're thinking it must be Vegetarian Times or New Age Journal right? Wrong! This was in *The Journal of the American Medical Association!* How about our war on cancer which is caused by the same big three foods? Here's what two time Nobel Prize winner Dr. Linus Pauling said:

"Everyone should know the war on cancer is largely a fraud."

George McGovern still chairmen of his commission called it a multibillion dollar medical failure."

The battle could be easily won but the consumer has to suffer because it is a huge business with huge profits with men running them that are determined to keep you unaware of their products' dangers. One of their goals is to keep the public thinking it's a bunch of tree huggers spreading propaganda instead of organizations like the prestigious *Advances in Cancer Research* that concluded:

"At present, we have overwhelming evidence...that none of the risk factors for cancer is....more significant than diet and nutrition."

The Senate itself wanted to know what the dietary influences are that promote cancer. The director of the National Cancer Institutes "Diet Nutrition and Cancer Program" Dr. Gio Gori reported:

"Until recently many eyebrows would have been raised by suggesting that an imbalance of normal dietary components could lead to cancer and cardiovascular disease....Today, the accumulation of evidence makes this notion not only possible, but CERTAIN...(The) dietary factors responsible (are) principally meat and fat intake."

---

[13] "Myths and Facts About Meat Production" displayed on National Cattlemen's Association website in 2001

The FTC, wanting an impartial expert to see if the same diets
that caused heart disease also caused cancer, called on a nutritional
scientist from Harvard, Dr. Mark Hegstead who testified.

"I think it is clear that the American diet is indicted as a cause of
coronary heart disease. And it is pertinent, I think, to point out
the same diet is now found 'Guilty' in terms of many forms of
cancer: breast cancer, cancer of the colon, and others..."

The bottom line is that today's factory animals are nothing like
the meats, eggs and dairy products of even 40 years ago. The
factory animals get no exercise and are fed with feed designed to
fatten them as rapidly and cheaply as possible. Even in 1975 at a
World Conference on Animal Production they announced the
remarkable finding that factory animals have as much as *30 times*
more saturated fat than yesterday's pasture-grazed animal did.
Instead of supplying the public with protein they are now
supplying us with saturated fat! As if that wasn't bad enough,
today's factory animals are subject to huge quantities of toxic
chemicals and artificial hormones. The residues are then consumed
by people that eat their flesh and drink their milk. Since most of
these pesticides, hormones, growth stimulants, insecticides,
tranquilizers, radioactive isotopes, herbicides, antibiotics and
larvacides didn't exist before World War II, we know little of their
long term health consequences though we do know they get in our
systems through the eating of the animals. We are now starting to
see some of those long-range results and they are unimaginable.

Beginning in the 1980's Dr. Saenz in Puerto Rico started
reporting one or two instances a day of young girls and boys only
four and five year old, that would be showing up with fully
developed breasts and ovarian cancers. She was quoted:

"I have seen hundreds of children like this, and I am certain
there are thousands more going undiagnosed because the
problem has become so widespread that many doctors are no
longer alarmed about it."

She described it as premature sexual development in the
February, 1982 *Journal of the Puerto Rico Medical Association*. She
went on to say:

"it was clearly related to local whole milk in the infant group. At a later age (the culprit was)... consumption of local whole milk, poultry and beef."

When asked how could she be so sure she responded simply: "when we take our patients off meat and fresh milk, their symptoms usually regress."[14]

Regulations in Puerto Rico are not as well enforced as in America so some of you might think that explains their epidemic but we're seeing more and more premature sexual development here as well. We're seeing much earlier puberty for both boys and girls with small children developing sexual characteristics and sexual aberrations. Sexual abuse of children has sky- rocketed and there are other indications that the human hormonal systems have gone haywire. When these hormones were first introduced after World War II, the meat industry was ecstatic and one manufacturer of DES called it the most important moment in the history of food production. It didn't take long before it was being used on 90% of the cattle to produce more fat and weight on the animals in the shortest possible amount of time. Meanwhile farmers that accidentally absorbed, inhaled or ingested even minute amounts of this "miracle drug" discovered something else all together.

"They exhibited symptoms of impotence, infertility, elevated and tender breasts or changes in voice register."[15]

Good God, what is going on? Later, a FDA biochemist Jackueline Verret was quoted saying "...it might be possible for only one molecule of DES in the 340 trillion present in a quarter pound of beef liver to trigger human cancer."[16]

After a fiercely fought political battle it was finally made illegal to administer DES to livestock. Did that stop the use? Hardly! The meat industry basically ignored this new law and several years after the ban, the FDA discovered more than half a million cattle that had been illegally implanted with the poison.[17] Even today many factory farms continue to use it and those that don't have switched

---

[14] Saenz de Rodriguez, Dr. C.A. "Journal of the Pourto Rico Medical Association" Feb. 1982
[15] Schell, O, "Modern Meat", Vintage Books, Random House
[16] Verrett, J. and Carper, J. "Eating May be Hazardous to your Helth" Simon and Schuster, 1974
[17] Schell, O. Ibid, page 198

to other sex hormones on the market that have much the same effect and contain many of the same ingredients. These hormones have names such as Steer-oid, Ralgro, Compudose and Synovex and are used in virtually every feedlot in the country.[18]

Still excited about having a steak for dinner?

Did you know the odds are you've been eating food nuked by irradiation whether you wanted to or not? You can thank the lobbying power of the meat industry for that one. For those that don't know what that means yet, it is the deliberate exposure of food to nuclear radiation in order to kill pathogens. This is the meat industry's answer to food-borne diseases. Their solution is not to clean up the filthy factory and slaughterhouse conditions they've created in search of the biggest profit, but to nuke them instead as it is a lot less expensive than changing the way they have to do business. As if that isn't scary enough, the meat industry lobbied aggressively so that foods that have been "nuked" wouldn't even have to be labeled at all, and if they did have to be labeled, they wanted the name changed to either "cold pasteurization" or "electron beam pasteurization."[19] Nice innocent sounding names for food that has been exposed to the equivalent of 2.5 million chest x-rays and already nicknamed the "food that will last forever."[20] Unfortunately on February, 22, 2000, the USDA legalized the irradiation of meat products and while a label is required on products sold in a store, no such luck for consumers at your local McDonald's, Burger King, or school cafeterias.[21] Actually, no such luck for any of the restaurants you might eat in for that matter!

The meat industry loves this new process because it supposedly kills the bacteria that creates E-coli contamination and other pathogens in animal products while not forcing them to clean up the environment in which the bacteria flourish. Most health-oriented organizations don't like it at all because they have no idea

---

[18] Ibid pgs. 257-268
[19] "Consumers and Companies Battle Over Meat Labels" Meat Industry Insights, May 29, 1999 and June 4, 1999
[20] Gibbs, Gary, "The Food That Would Last Forever" Avery Publishing, 1993
[21] Ibid note 52, page 40

of the long-term results of what that nuclear radiation can do to people over the long haul. There have been short-term studies, however, so we do know that irradiating food destroys vitamins A, C, E. K and B-1 while forming new and potentially carcinogenic chemical compounds.[22] Plus there is the very real possibility that it could create mutant bacteria and viruses.[23] I guess the meat industry figures they'll worry about that when they have to. Here's what John Gofman, M.D., professor emeritus of molecular and cell biology, professor at University of California School of Medicine and founder of the Biomedical Research Division at Livermore National Laboratory had to say on the subject:

"Food irradiation causes a host of unnatural and unidentifiable chemicals to be formed within the irradiated foods. Our ignorance about these foreign compounds makes it simply a fraud to tell the public 'we know' irradiated foods would be safe to eat. It is dishonorable to talk people into buying irradiated foods."[24]

On August 10, 2000 Reuters News Service released a report that said:

"A report by the United States Department of Agriculture estimates that 89% of U.S. beef ground into patties contains traces of the deadly E.coli strain."[25]

So how wide spread is the use of hormones in US beef production? It's more than 90% overall and 100% in the larger feedlots.[26] U.S. cattlemen keep trying to convince the public that they're safe. My question becomes, if that's true, then why since 1995 has the European Union prohibited treating any farm animal with sex hormones to promote growth? Their studies have revealed that they are *known* to cause several human cancers and reproductive dysfunction.[27] They went so far as to refuse any of the hormone-treated meat being shipped in from America. It's interesting how the U.S. meat industry responded to the Europeans' refusal. First they tried to use tariffs to ram our meat

[22] Robbins, J. "Diet Revolution"
[23] Robbins John, "Diet Revolution"
[24] quoted in Gillete, Becky, "Try Our Nukeburgers," July/August 2000
[25] Karleff, Ian, "Canadian Scientists Test E-coli Vaccine on Source, Reuters News Service, Aug.10, 2000
[26] Fox, Spoiled
[27] Ibid. page 179

down their throats.[28] When that didn't work we went and
complained to the World Trade Organization (WTO) who ruled
the European Union was required to pay the United States
$150,000,000 per year as compensation for lost profits. They
issued that ruling despite a long report by independent scientists
showing some hormones added to U.S. meat are "completely
carcinogen" – capable of causing cancer by themselves.[29] Do you
not find it a bit ominous that the health risks from U.S. beef are so
enormous that the Europeans are willing to pay 150 million a year
rather than allow our beef to cross their borders?[30]

All you ex-smokers, have I got your attention yet?

Let's look at some other fall-outs from this industry. It would be
almost impossible to overestimate the impact that cattle grazing is
having on this country. 70% of all the western land area is
presently being used for grazing. More than two-thirds of the entire
land area of Montana, Wyoming, Colorado, New Mexico, Arizona,
Nevada, Utah, and Idaho is used for grazing. That's roughly 525
million acres, nearly 2 acres for every person in the U.S. Yet, almost
all the land is publicly owned. That's right, it belongs to you and
future generations. Right now 70% of all the land in western
national forests and 90% of the Bureau of Land Management land
are grazed by livestock for private profit! Let's use New Mexico for
one detailed example.[31]

Amount paid by New Mexico's Governor in 1994 to graze his
cattle on 17,000 acres of trust land – 65 cents an acre.

Amount paid by New Mexico's 1994 candidate for Land
Commissioner Stirling Spencer to graze his cattle on 20,000 acres
of trust land – 59 cents an acre.

Amount New Mexico livestock ranchers do not pay in property
taxes, sales tax, or other taxes due to special deductions and
exemptions given to the cattle industry – Billions of dollars
annually!

[28] Barnard, Neal, "The Power of Your Plate" (Summertown, TN: Book Publishing Co. 1990)
[29] Ibid. page 165
[30] Robbins, John – all notes 57-61 on page 143, "Diet Revolution"
[31] Robbins John

Number of states with higher taxes on the poor than New
Mexico – 3

Number of states with a greater percentage of women living in
poverty – 0

Here's another side effect of eating from the American
slaughterhouse that most people don't realize. Because the meat
industry has been constantly feeding antibiotics to the livestock,
we're now to the point where many disease-producing organisms
are becoming increasingly resistant to antibiotics. For instance just a
few years ago less than 10% of the staphylococci bacteria
(notorious for skin, bone and wound infections as well as
pneumonia and food poisoning) were resistant to penicillin. Now
over 90% of staphylococci are resistant to penicillin. John Robbins
reminds us:

> "It is no exaggeration to say that the indiscriminate use of
> antibiotics in factory farms is systematically producing disease
> causing agents that are invulnerable to the modern wonder drugs.
> To keep the animals alive under such horrid conditions,
> antibiotics are, as a matter of course, placed in their feed. This use
> of substances which are responsible for so many medical miracles
> is creating an "anti-miracle."[32]

Even though Great Britain and the European Economic
Community forbade the chronic use of antibiotics in the livestock
feed in their countries, the pharmaceutical and livestock industries
here in America have successfully defeated every single attempt to
follow suit in the U.S.

Did you know the livestock population in America consumes
enough grain and soybeans to feed the entire human population of
America 5 times over?[33] They eat 80% of the corn we grow and
over 95% of the oats.[34] In return for this inefficient use of acreage
we get one pound of meat on our plates for every 16 pounds of
grain we feed the animals. The other 15 pounds becomes manure
which then gets washed into our water supply polluting yet another

---

[32] Robbins, J, "Diet For A New America"
[33] Bralove, Mary, "The Food Crisis" Wall Street Journal, Oct.3, 1974
[34] Maidenburg, H.J. "The Livestock Population Explosion" New York Times July 1,
   1973, pg. 1 Finance section

precious resource. Meanwhile, the Institute for Food and
Development policy tells us that 40,000 children starve to death on
this planet every day.

Let's put it another way. To supply one person with a meat habit
for a year requires 3¼ acres of land. A pure vegetarian requires 1/6
of an acre. That would mean we could feed 20 more people in a
much healthier fashion, while not polluting our world beyond
repair.[35] Lester Brown of the Overseas Development Council
estimated if Americans were to reduce their meat consumption by
only 10% it would free up 12 million tons of grain annually for
human consumption. That by itself would be enough to adequately
feed every single one of the 60 million humans who will starve to
death this year.[36]

Just the world's cattle consumption alone, not to mention pigs
and chickens, consume a quantity of food equal to the caloric needs
of 8.7 billion people – nearly double the entire human population
of the planet.[37] Here's yet another way of looking at it, this time
according to the Dept. of Agriculture. One acre of land can
produce 20,000 pounds of potatoes as opposed to 165 pounds of
beef.[38]

One question often brought up by those pushing meat that does
deserve attention, is the question of where does one get their
vitamin B-12 as that is necessary for proper health. Also they say,
"if vegetarian is such a healthy way of eating why doesn't nature
provide vitamin B-12 elsewhere besides meat?" The fact is, it used
to when we could drink the water from our steams and our water
supply wasn't contaminated and now chlorinated. You'd also have
been getting it from the grooves of carrots and the skin of potatoes
from the earth, but all the chemical fertilizers have put an end to
that. The recommended dietary allowance of vitamin B-12 is
incredibly tiny, just 2 millionths of a gram but it is necessary now
for vegans to make sure they get it in a multi-vitamin. The other

[35] Lappe, Francis Moore, Diet For a Small Planet, Ballantine Books, N.Y. 1982
[36] Rensberger, Boyce, "Curb on U.S. Waste Urged to Help World Hunger" New York
Times, Oct. 25, 1974
[37] Rensberger, Boyce, New York Times article, Nov. 5, 1974
[38] ibid. 68

important nutrient that our bodies need, is the Omega 3 fats. The reality is you'd have to eat 20 supermarket eggs to get as much Omega –3 that is provided in one egg from a free range chicken.[39] They are plentiful in flax seed oil, fatty fish such as salmon, herring and sardines, and can be found in walnuts and green leafy vegetables as well. It's now being discovered that flax seed oil has many advantages over the fish oils.

Most of us heard about the cattlemen taking Oprah Winfrey to court and suing her for $600,000 for her comments about not eating meat once she learned cattle byproducts were being fed back to the cattle as feed, literally turning them into cannibals. This is the practice that leads to what is commonly known as Mad Cow Disease. Millions of cattle in Europe have had to be destroyed because of this practice and its nightmarish symptoms. In the suit against Oprah it claimed that one of her guests was allowed to "present biased, unsubstantiated and irresponsible claims against beef" and went on to say that doing so "goes beyond all possible bounds of decency and is utterly intolerable in a civilized community."[40]

The court found instead, that the opinions had been based on "truthful, established facts." They also pointed out that the opinions on which they had been sued were almost identical to a report the FDA released nine months after the lawsuit had begun. One part of the story that didn't get much exposure was what Oprah said on the courthouse steps after the verdict:

"I'm still never going to eat another burger."

Some more meat industry propaganda that should be pointed out is the meat industries' tenacity in asserting that children must have meat in order to have proper brain development, telling us:

"Consuming 2-3 servings a day of the meat group is important to achieve cognitive brain function."[41]

When you compare that comment, with all the scientific data we

[39] Simpoulos, Artemis and Robinson. The omega Diet: The Life Saving Nutrional Diet of Crete, Harper, 1999
[40] Petition by Paul Engler and Cactus Feeders against Oprah Winfrey, U.S. District Court, Texas, May 28, 1996
[41] "Meats Nutients and Cognitive Development" Facts from the Meat Board; Nutrition, 1995

now have available it is quite a remarkable statement. One such study published in the *Journal of the American Dietetic Association* found that whereas the I.Q. of the average U.S. child is 99, the average I.Q. of the vegetarian child was 116.[42] Here's what one of the most brilliant minds of our century, Albert Einstein, had to say on the subject:

> *"Nothing will benefit human health and increase the chances for survival on earth as much as the evolution to a vegetarian diet."*

So who are you gonna believe, an unbiased observer like Einstein, reminding us that evolution is about evolving beyond the meat-eating state of consciousness most of us have been stuck in, or the people who make their living from selling you their dead food products? In 2000 the Public Health Institute released a major study that found fully a third of all today's teens could face:

> "chronic and debilitating health problems" such as diabetes, heart disease and cancer *by their early thirties.*[43]

"The Sky Is Falling, The Sky Is Falling"
– Chicken Little

So what comes first, the truth about the chicken or the eggs they've been laying? I hate to tell you this, but the reality is almost everything that's going on with the factory animals in the beef industry applies to the poultry industry as well, only in greater numbers as a lot more people eat chicken than beef. The chickens raised for meat are called broilers and it is a mammoth industry. Approximately eight billion broilers are killed each year in the United States for food – a number larger than the population of the entire planet.[44]

To give you an idea of what you're eating, traditionally it took a broiler 21 weeks to reach the desired four pound market weight; now since they're being bred with hormones it only takes seven

---

[42] Dwyer, J.T. "Mental Age and IQ of predominatly Vegetarian Children" Journal of ADS, 1980:
[43] Coleman, Jennifer, "Soft Drink Firms Defend Contracts" Santa Cruz Sentinel, Sept. 27, 2000, C-2
[44] USDA National Statistics Service, "Facts About the Poultry Industry" Animal Protection Institute

weeks to reach the same weight. Lancaster Farming put it into a perspective that certainly caught my attention:

> "If a seven pound human baby grew at the same rate of today's turkeys and chickens, when the baby reached 18 weeks of age it would weigh 1,500 pounds."[45]

Ninety percent of broiler chickens are so obese by 6 weeks they can't even walk. The conditions where they are bred are so disgusting and horrendous it's hard for most people to even imagine. It's interesting that as more and more of the public is discovering these disgusting inhumane conditions, the chicken factories are using words like natural, hormone-free, organic, and vegetarian on their labels. The reality is they're "just hoodwinking the public" says Allen Shainsky, developer of Rocky the Range Chicken. He goes on to add:

> "right now anyone can say almost anything on a label about their chicken …. conventional chicken can even use the word 'natural.' " [46]

He goes on to say that basically the federal law is toothless and poultry companies use 'free range' strictly as a marketing gimmick. There is no law or regulation defining what is "free range," so unless you know the owner personally or at least can trust the word of your health food store owner who knows the farmer personally, I'd avoid chickens altogether.

Let's look at the other end of the chicken industry and see how honest they've been with the public. The egg industry ran a series of ads in the Wall Street Journal that the American Heart Association took issue with because it claimed:

> "there is no scientific evidence that eating eggs, even in quantity, will increase the risk of a heart attack."

The American Heart Association then went to the FTC to prohibit this "false, deceptive and misleading advertising" so the egg industry hired the best legal counsel it could find and they took it to court. After hearing all the arguments from both sides, this was part of the judge's 101 page decision in which he not only agreed it was "false, misleading and deceptive" but wrote:

---

[45] Quoted in "Birds Exploited for Meat" Farm Sanctuary, May 26, 1997
[46] Bjerklie, Steve, "Fowl Play" Sonoma County Independent/Metro Active, May 15, 1997

"There exists a substantial body of competent and reliable scientific evidence that eating eggs increases the risk of heart attacks or heart disease…" then he goes on to add "This evidence is systematic, consistent, strong and congruent."[47]

As reported in *The Journal of the American Medical Association*, The Center for Disease Control and Prevention now strongly advises consumers "to avoid recipes using raw eggs."[48] In fact, many egg based foods that were consumed in the past are now considered by the CDC to be unsafe to eat, due to the salmonella contamination that is so widespread. These include soft boiled, poached, sunny-side up, Caesar salads, homemade eggnog, lemon meringue pie, Hollandaise sauce, raw cookie dough, and several classic types of cake frosting.[49]

The egg industry still keeps trying to deny the link between eggs and heart disease. When the Senate Select Committee on Nutrition and Human Needs met to establish guidelines for the nation's food choices, the egg industry presented five different research studies they claimed exonerated eggs. They were so confusing that the chairman of the commission, George McGovern, asked the National Heart Lung and Blood Institute for an expert opinion on their validity. After the institute carefully examined all five studies they reported to Congress that *the studies seemed deliberately designed to "distort the facts."* The institute's impartial appraisal was that the studies were:

"seriously flawed….meaningless and should be discarded."

Did this give the industry pause? Hardly! The false advertising continued unabated. In fact, even more so as they inserted millions of flyers into egg cartons reassuring consumers that "eggs don't raise cholesterol."

What You Don't Know Could Kill Both You And Your Children

Let's move on to some other areas that should be of concern to

---

[47] "Orders a Stop on Egg Claims" New York Daily News, Dec 12, 1975, pg. 62
[48] "The Emergence of Grade A Eggs as a Major Source of Samonella Infections" Journal of AMA 25,1988
[49] Fox, "Spoiled"

you. Did you know the average American child sees 1,000 ads a week promoting sugared cereals, sodas, candy and other junk food so they are totally addicted by the time they reach their teen years? More than 5,000 schools in the US now have contracts with fast food companies and junk food manufacturers to provide food for their cafeterias and/or vending machines.[50] Coca Cola along with others are giving millions to cash strapped schools for exclusive rights to sell their products in our schools.[51] Today the average North American consumes, per day, 53 teaspoons of sugar – *that amounts to a five pound bag of sugar every 10 days for each man, woman, and child.*[52] And we wonder why obesity is now the number one killer?

As if it's not bad enough, these industries push their food like a drug dealer pushes drugs inflicting incalculable damage on our country. Baskin Robbins now has more ice cream stores in Tokyo than in Los Angeles and Mexico has now surpassed the US. in per capita consumption of Coca Cola.[53] As John Robbins so diplomatically puts it:

"In light of this, the meat, dairy and egg industries have done the only thing they could. They have joined hands with the tobacco industry to do whatever they can to confuse the issue and make the public think 'anything can cause cancer.' They figure the more people that think anything can cause cancer, the less they are to focus on those *specific things which in fact are known to cause cancer.* It's not that these industries want people to get cancer; it's just that they want us to continue buying their products. *The fact that their products do, in fact, cause cancer, is in their minds, a deeply unfortunate public relations issue.*"

Folks, this so called public relations issue is not only causing heart disease and cancer but many other diseases that have also been traced directly to today's dietary blindness. Here's just a short list you might consider before eating that next hamburger, fried chicken or making your child drink three glasses of milk a day:

---

[50] Gardner, Gary Halweil, Brian, "Escaping Hunger, Escaping Excess" WorldWatch, July /August 2000
[51] Ibid.
[52] Robbins, John, "The Revolution Diet"
[53] Gardner and Halweil, "Escaping Hunger"

Diabetes: Millions of Americans who suffer from this disease do not know their agony could be greatly reduced and in many cases even eliminated entirely by different diet choices. In *Lancet,* Dr. Inder Singh reported a study in which 80 diabetic patients were restricted to very low-fat diets and forbidden any sugar consumption. Within six weeks over 60% of the patients no longer required insulin. In the next few weeks that number rose to 70% and those who still required insulin needed only a fraction of what they had required before the diet change. The *American Journal of Clinical Nutrition* reported a study in which 20 diabetics were put on a high fiber very low-fat diet. After only 16 days, 45% of the patients were able to get off insulin altogether. Other studies have confirmed that 75% of diabetics who needed insulin and 90% of diabetics who needed pills can be freed of their medication in a matter of weeks on a low-fat high fiber diet.

Hypoglycemia: Excess fat is just as much to blame as sugar. Again a low-fat natural diet can do wonders.

Multiple Sclerosis: Most people would be astounded if they knew some of the nutritional research on this "incurable" disease. Dr. Roy Swank, head of the Department of Neurology at University of Oregon began treating "incurable" patients on a natural low fat, low protein diet staying away from meat and dairy and monitored them for 20 years. Almost 90% *(ninety percent)* who began the low-fat diet during the early stages of the disease not only arrested the process, but actually improved over the next 20 years. Of those victims that began the diet at an intermediate stage of the disease, over 65% were able to prevent further damage. Even more amazing is that even 30% of the victims that began the low-fat diet when the disease was well advanced were able to arrest the devastation and showed no further decline. Over the last 35 years, Dr. Swank treated several thousand M.S. patients and found that those who discovered it early stood a 95% chance of arresting it, and for many there is a very real possibility of a cure." All because of the natural low fat diet off of both milk and meat.

Ulcers: There has been a lot of study done on this malady as it has become so common, but by and large the public has no idea that ulcers occur most often and most severely in diets that are low in fiber, high in fat and acid forming. There are powerful economic interests that would prefer you don't know that. In case you've forgotten, meats, eggs and fish are the most acid forming of all the foods. For many years however, this is one of the few things that milk was actually considered to be good for. We now know differently. Though milk does offer temporary relief from the pain by neutralizing the acids, they now know it often makes matters worse as milk increases natural acid production. They have discovered that cabbage, broccoli, cauliflower, mustard greens, kale and collards contain a substance so effective for ulcers that it is nicknamed "Vitamin U."[54] Also I found of great interest that the simple act of "chewing one's food" is very important to the treatment of ulcers as human saliva is highly alkaline while people who don't chew well are actually setting themselves up for problems down the road.

Arthritis: At Wayne State University Medical School a few medical researchers went out on a limb and went against everything the Arthritis Foundation said about the correlation between diet and arthritis and put six rheumatoid arthritic patients on a fat free diet. In seven weeks time all the patients had lost all their symptoms. Then when fats were reintroduced into their diets within three days their symptoms reappeared.[55] I find it startling that this isn't common knowledge yet. We now know in parts of the world where diets are low in fat and cholesterol, moderate in protein and where processed food is minimal, that even the old people that have done hard physical labor their entire lives are basically arthritis free.[56] Bottom line is that there is plenty of evidence that strongly suggests diets very low in saturated fat, low in protein and high in fiber, without any cholesterol, would be best in the prevention and treatment of arthritis. I daresay it's no wonder the meat, dairy and poultry industries would prefer if this wasn't common knowledge.

[54] Hut, R. "Food Reform: Our Desperate Need," Neidkebburg Publishers, 1975
[55] Lucas, P., "Dietary Fat Aggravates Active Rheumatoid Sarthritis" Clinical Research, 29:754A, 1981
[56] Valkenburg, H. "Osteoarthritis in Some Developing Countries" Journal of Rheumatology, 10:20, 1983; Soloman, L. "Rheumatic Disorders in the South African Negro" South African Medical Journal, 49:1292, 1975; Beasley, R. "Low Prevalence of Rheumatoid Arthritis in Chinese..." Journal of Rheumatology, 10:11 1983

Kidney Stones: Rather than repeat myself I'd rather refer you back for more detail to John Robbins *Diet for a New America,* but suffice it to say that 99% of all kidney stones can be prevented by a low protein, high fiber, low-fat diet with no cholesterol.[57] The more animal protein we eat the more calcium our kidneys have to excrete. Vegetarians who still eat dairy and eggs in the U.S. have fewer than half the kidney stones of the general population,[58] while pure vegetarians have almost none.

Gallstones: The main ingredient in gallstones is cholesterol. World wide they have found the greatest incidence of gallbladder disease, gallstones and gallbladder cancer is in people whose food choices are low in fiber, high in cholesterol and fat – in other words, your typical American diet.[59] Low-fat, high fiber diets not only prevent gallstones, they often can relieve the pain so significantly they make surgery unnecessary for people that already have them.[60]

High Blood Pressure: More visits to the doctor and more prescriptions are written each year for this ailment than any other disease[61] – in other words there are huge financial incentives involved in the treatment of this form of distress. In countries where the intake of salt, fats and cholesterol is low, high blood pressure is virtually non-existent.[62] They live instead on whole grains, fresh fruit and vegetables and eat very little processed food. Many people in their 80's have the same blood pressure as teenagers. By the way, these are the same countries where strokes and heart attacks are few and far between.

In laymen terms, high blood pressure is a warning to you that your circulatory system is not well. This should be considered a fire

[57] Derrick, F. "Kidney Stone Disease: Evaluation and Medical Management," Postgraduate Medical Journal, 66:115, 1979

[58] Robertson, W. "Dietary Changes and the Incidence of Urinary Calculi... Journal of Chronic Diseases, 32:469, 1979

[59] Hill, M., "Colon Cancer and Diet with Special Reference to Intakes of Fat and Fiber" American Journal of Clinical Nutrition, 29:1417,1976

[60] Boston Collaborative Drug Surveillance Program, "Surgically Confirmed Gallbladder Disease...New England Journal of Medicine, 290:15, 1974

[61] Baum, C., "Drug Use in the United States In 1981," Journal of the American Medial Association, 25:1293, 1984

[62] Freis, E. "Salt, Volume and the Prevention of Hypertension" Circulation, 53-589, 1976 Editorial "Why Does Blood Pressure Rise With Age"

alarm calling for immediate attention. Unfortunately, the conventional response is to silence the alarm with drugs while doing little about what set off the alarm in the first place. These drugs also have many side effects that cause other problems. Doesn't it make a lot more sense if the focus instead was on teaching people to change their diets where they can accomplish the same results without all the side effects? The drugs certainly have a part to play as they can bring down the pressure, but our doctors should be telling you how to eat so you don't get the high pressure in the first place. I don't need to remind you that the drug industry has tremendous power in this country just like the meat and dairy industries.

So what is the proper diet? This is easy to know since the same foods that raise blood cholesterol also raise blood pressure. Did you know cheese is among the highest foods in salt content? Unfortunately for the US public, the dairy industry is so strong they can confuse the issue for many people with their advertising and lobbying clout in Washington. Also, the dairy industry is the second largest seller of saturated fats by the way, coming in second behind guess who? The meat industry. So now we have all the hundreds of billions of dollars and clout of the drug, dairy and meat industries all with a vested interest in keeping the public in the dark. The problem is we live in a drug-oriented culture fond of instant results. If you come up with a drug that lowers your blood pressure you'll make lots of money, but showing people how to eat so it never gets elevated in the first place is a contrary action not likely to be high on their list of priorities. So the elite few that run the "Great American Food Machine" keep getting rich at the expense of the ill-informed public because they can throw a lot of money into advertising and confuse the truth. At this very moment millions of people are suffering from having high blood pressure related disorders. "This is especially tragic because it is so thoroughly needless."[63]

Asthma: Researchers at the University Hospital in Linkoping, Sweden, put severe bronchial asthma patients on a pure vegetarian diet without eggs or dairy. After one year on the diet, more than 90% of the patients reported a major improvement in not only

[63] Robbins, J. "Diet For a New America"

severity but number of asthma attacks. Level of medication
dropped an average of 50-90% and a number of patients were so
improved that they were able to discontinue medication altogether
with the pure vegetarian diet.[64]

There is so much data available about the pork and veal
industries as well as enormous amount of data about dozens of
other diseases but I think you get the picture. We need to ask
ourselves, all this is for what? So we can devour dead animals that
will eventually ravage our bodies and turn them into "tombs" as
Jesus called it?"

Rachel Carson wrote a book called *Silent Spring* in memory of
the song birds that have begun to disappear from our world.[65] I
believe it should be required reading in all our high schools. The
reason the song birds are the first to die off from all these
chemicals, she explains, is that they are at the top of long food
chains. As one organism eats another they build up in higher and
higher concentrations. A bird ingests the pesticides of all the tens of
thousands of worms it has eaten. A larger fish will accumulate in its
body the total amount of poisons accumulated by the thousands of
smaller fish it eats.

By the same token a cow or chicken or pig will retain in its flesh
all the pesticides it has ever eaten as well, and they build up rather
fast for a number of reasons. First, they are fed great quantities of
fish-meal as it is cheap. Secondly, their other feeds are grown on
lands that have been heavily sprayed. Thirdly, they are dipped,
sprayed and fed many toxic compounds they would never
encounter were they raised in a more natural way. These poisons
are all retained in the fat of the animals which the unsuspecting
public eventually eats. Recent studies show that of all the toxic
chemical residues in the American diet, 95-99% comes from meat,
fish, dairy products and eggs.[66]

Here's what the EPA had to say:

---

[64] Lindahl, O., "Vegan Regimen with Reduced Medication in the Treatment of
Bronchial Asthma" Journal of Asthma, 22:24, 1985
[65] Carson, R. Silent Spring, Crest Books, 1962
[66] Harris, S. "Organochlorine Contamination of Breast Milk" Environmental
Defense Fund, Washington D.C.

"Foods of animal origin are the major source of....pesticide residues in the diet,"[67]

Remember Agent Orange from Vietnam that turned out to be so devastating to our veterans later on? Well two of its active ingredients 2,4-D and 2,4,5-T are sprayed on land used to grow feed for our livestock. Millions of pounds are used even though one particular substance found in 2,4,5-T is so toxic DDT looks like a "glass of champagne" in comparison says Robbins.

When referring to Dioxin, the head of Toxic Effects Branch of the EPA's National Environmental Research Center, Dr. Diane Courtney called it

"...by far the most toxic chemical known to mankind."[68]

The EPA has recognized that cattle which graze on land sprayed with 2,4,5-T accumulate Dioxin in their fat.[69] Dow Chemical on the other hand who profits greatly from sales of this poison says

"...2,4,5-T is about as toxic as aspirin."

Here's a couple quick statistics that I found quite revealing as to the job our protection agencies are doing on our behalf. The USDA tests only one out of every 250,000 slaughtered animals for toxic chemical residues and even then it tests for only 10% of the toxic chemicals known to be in our meat supply.[70] So low are our standards that inspectors from the European Economic Community (EEC) declared 11 of the largest meat packers ineligible to export their products through the Common Market. [71]

I'll close this section for now with a story that dramatizes the relationship between meat and toxic chemicals that would be hilarious if it weren't the truth. On April 5, 1973 the EPA finally banned the artificial coloring agent Violet 1 as a carcinogen. Up until that very day the Department of Agriculture had been using the dye to stamp meats with the grades of "Choice", "Prime", and

[67] Duggan, R. "Dietary Intake of Pesticide Chemicals in the U.S., June 1966-April 1968" Pesticide Monitoring Journal, 2:140-52, 1969
[68] Courtney, Dr D. testimony before Senate Commerce Committee on the Environment, August 9, 1974
[69] Federal Register, Dec 13, 1979, pg. 72, 325
[70] "Mainstream", Summer 1983, pg.17
[71] "U.S. Meat Banned for Export Through the Common Market," Vegetarian Times, Oct. 1984, pg.17

"U.S. No.1 USDA." *For over 20 years the USDA had been reassuring customers that their meat was healthy by stamping it with a cancer causing dye.* I must say, "I'm certainly reassured!"

So You Want To Be A Parent?

I would be remiss to not repeat this EPA statistic for all the women of child bearing age. They analyzed the breast milk of vegetarian women and discovered the levels of pesticides in their milk was far less than the average. A later study published in the *New England Journal of Medicine* found:

"The highest level of contamination in the breast milk of the vegetarian was lower than the lowest level in non-vegetarian women... The mean vegetarian levels were only one or two percent as high as the average in the United States."[72]

And this is for vegetarians that still drink milk – the average for women that are pure vegetarian is probably significantly even better. The mothers of the future might want to take this to heart.

For all you men who may one day want to father a child, we now know without a doubt the gene pool is being adversely affected. That is why the offspring of Vietnam veterans affected with Agent Orange have such a high rate of birth defects and why a University of Southern California Medical School study found distinct correlation between brain tumors in children, and their fathers' exposure to toxic chemicals.[73]

I find it hard to not feel enraged at those who are lying and profiting from such abominations. Unfortunately, at this point in history, since it is greed that rules our society as well as our government, a guy like Paul Oreffice, the President of Dow Chemical Company can get on NBC's Today show and lull people to sleep with comments like:

"there's absolutely no evidence of dioxin doing any damage to humans."

He said this despite knowing that the amount of dioxin sufficient to kill 10 million people could fit in a space smaller than a human hand.[74]

---

[72] March 26, 1981 "New England Journal of Medicine"
[73] Hilts, P., "Chemicals at Parent's Job May Cause Child's Tumor" Washington Post, July 3, 1981
[74] Robbins, J., "Diet For a New America"

America's Most Precious Resource

Another disaster looming from our addiction to meat and the meat industry's abuse of our land, is that we are eliminating possibly our most precious natural resource, topsoil, at an unbelievable rate. Two hundred years ago most of our cropland had at least 21 inches of topsoil. We're down below 6 inches at this point and accelerating fast.[75] The U.S. Department of Agriculture says that our productivity is down 70%, with much of our land on the brink of becoming barren wasteland.[76] The USDA even admits this is an unparalleled disaster in the making, but claims that: "...halting soil erosion and degradation would be prohibitively expensive."[77] The U.S. Soil Conservation Service reports our topsoil loss amounts to 7 billion tons a year or 4 million acres.[78] Folks, that's about the size of Connecticut. Of this incredible loss, 85% is directly associated with the raising of life stock.[79]

As Robbins puts it, "Without a major change in what we consume for nutrition we are well on our way to losing what many scientists feel has always been the basis of our strength as a nation. If the present pace of soil erosion continues, it is just a matter of time until the people of the US, the inheritors of the world's richest farmlands, will be forced to depend on foreign imports for food."[80]

A vegetarian life style on the other hand makes less than 5% of the demand on our soil as meat-oriented choices.[81] Here are some revealing numbers to consider next time you buy a hamburger from McDonald's:

U.S. corn eaten by people – 2%

U.S. corn eaten by livestock – 77%

[75] Hur, Robin, "Six Inches from Starvation; How and why America's Topsoil is Disappearing" Vegetarian Times, March 1985
[76] Brune, William, State Soil Conservationist Des Moines, Iowa in testimony before Senate Committee on Agriculture and Forestry, July 6, 1976
[77] Cited in Hur, as per note 72
[78] Ibid.
[79] Soil and Water Conservation Act – Summary of Appraisal, USDA Review Draft, 1980, pg.18;USDA, Economics and Statistics Service, Natural Resource Capital in US Agriculture Irrigation, Drainage and Conservation Investments Since 1900, ESCS Staff Paper, March, 1979
[80] Robbins, J. "Diet For a New America"
[81] Ibid. note 68

U.S. farmland producing vegetables – 4 million acres
U.S. farmland producing hay for livestock – 56 million acres
U.S. grain and cereals fed to livestock – 70%
Human Beings who could be fed by the grain and soybeans eaten
by U.S. livestock – 1.4 billion
World's population living in the U.S. – 4%
World's beef eaten in the U.S. – 23%[82]
Did you know our current agricultural system, which is designed
to feed America's meat habit, wastes almost all the food it grows by
feeding it to livestock. This creates a constant pressure to get the
highest yield out of the land whatever the ecological cost. As a
result, we have lost hundreds of millions of acres to soil erosion.
Last count was 260 million acres of forest that had been
converted.[83] Since 1967, that rate of deforestation has been about
an acre every five seconds (an area the size of a football field every
second.)[84] By comparison for every acre that is converted for
homes, roads, shopping centers etc., seven acres are lost converting
land into grazing for livestock or growing livestock feed. Forests, by
the way, just happen to be one of the few places where topsoil
erosion doesn't occur.

Extinction Means Forever

Here's another little known fact worth pondering. Since 1960
when the US began to import meat, Central America was blessed
with 130,000 square miles of virgin rainforest. We've already
destroyed over half (and that's the conservative estimate) so
Americans can have seemingly cheap hamburgers. By the way, it's
worth noting these rainforests are among the world's most precious
natural resources. The rainforests contain 80% of the earth's land
vegetation which accounts
for a large percentage of our oxygen. Did you know America is the
only country in the world to not agree to do something about

[82] All these statistics found in John Robbins "The Food Revolution"
[83] Hur, Robin, "Are High Fat Diets Killing our Forests?" Vegetarian Times, Feb. 1984
[84] "Livestock and Environment" Agriculture 21, Agriculture Dept. Food and Agriculture Organization, United Nations

global warning? Here's part of a letter sent to our president from 49 Nobel Prize-winning scientists 12 years ago:

"Global warming has emerged as the most serious environmental threat of the 21st century....only by taking action now can we assure that future generations will not be put at risk."[85]

Do you know how absurd this is when you consider what we're destroying in return for a habit that is literally killing us, costing us hundreds of billions in health costs, and ruining the environment for future generations? Lee Iaccoco summed up beautifully the corporate and governmental mindset concerning this looming tragedy.

"We've got to pause and ask ourselves: How much clean air do we need?" ...and this is one of our corporate leaders? Obviously we can't look there for help.

Did you know that even though a third of Costa Rica is already being used to raise cattle, the remainder of that tiny country still houses more bird species than all of the U.S. combined?[86]

With the hamburgerization of the Central American rainforests, many of our migratory birds are losing their winter homes and are dying. Not only do we lose their beauty but they play a major role in keeping the insect population of America down. So to make up for it, we must increase our use of pesticides which end up getting into our food chain, thereby polluting our bodies even more. What a vicious cycle we have created all for the sake of cheap hamburgers. Folks, it's just not that hard to understand. If you're wondering why doesn't our government put a stop to it, I'll tell you why – because the same corporate interests are in bed with the politicians on both the local and national level and that's what gets them elected. (For those of you interested, I've come up with some creative solutions to that problem in my new book *You May Be Right, but CONSIDER THIS...* – Musings of a Spiritual Truckdriver Fasting From Ignorance.

Add to that scenario that the current rate of extinction in the

[85] Booth, W. "Action Urged Against Global Warning; Scientists Appeal for Curbs on Gases" Washington Post, Feb.2, 1990
[86] Acres, U.S.A., Kansas City, Missouri, Volume 15, No.6, June 1985, pg. 2

world is 1000 species per year and the rate is accelerating rapidly. At the rate we're going in the next 30 years over a million species will become extinct.[87] What a travesty is being done by the meat industry when we know so little about the natural resources of these rainforests. We do know their preservation is essential to the ecology of the world as we're just discovering that in those forests are the insects that could very well supplant pesticides for controlling insect pests back here at home. Already, 25% of all our medicines are derived from raw materials that are found in these forests. A child suffering from Leukemia now has an 80% chance of survival as opposed to a 20% chance, thanks to a rainforest plant called the rosy periwinkle.

At this point less than 1% of the plant species of these rainforests have been tested for medicinal benefits and we're wiping them out at an average of one species an hour. *ONE SPECIES AN HOUR!* [88] To add insult to injury, we now know the damage is irreparable since the rapidly growing trees and plants of the rainforests have consumed almost all the minerals from the soil, unlike our Northern forests where much remains in the ground. As a result, once the land is cleared, vegetation has an extra hard time growing back at all. Also, with the removal of the plant cover, the hard rains there cause extremely rapid soil erosion. Immediately after clearing, it takes two and a half acres to support one steer, but within a few short years the land has become so eroded it takes 12 acres! In 10 years after that *one* steer may require as much as *20 acres* of land.[89]

So let me repeat this in other words – *our meat habit is turning lush rainforests with countless untapped resources that are one of the earth's few remaining treasures into deserts, useless even for grazing by the cattle they were destroyed to feed.*

I'm sorry, but that's just plain obscene by any stretch of the imagination. Ask yourself, "is a pound of hamburger worth half a ton of Brazilian rainforest? Is 67 square feet of rainforest – an area the size of one small kitchen – too much to pay for one hamburger? These and other similar questions are being asked too little and too

[87] ibid.
[88] Robbins J, "Diet For a New America"
[89] Ibid.

late to preserve much of the great tropical rainforest of the Amazon, and its environment. It took nature thousands of years to form the rainforest, but it took a mere 25 years for people to destroy much of it. And the real bottom line we need to look at is, *when rainforest is gone, it's gone forever."* [90]

Our Other Greatest Resource

Now how about our other greatest resource, water? Many say that water will be more expensive than oil within our own lifetimes, and when you look at the fact many people pay a $1.50 for a liter of bottled water in America now....hmmm – gas is how much for a gallon? It looks like it's already proving to be true. By the way, many parts of the world have almost no clean drinking water already.

Here's a quote from Newsweek magazine:

"The water that goes into a 1,000 pound steer would float a destroyer."

An older estimate had it that a single pound of meat takes over 2,500 gallons of water, which is as much as a typical family uses for all its combined household purposes in a month.[91] What most people don't realize are the huge economic costs to the average taxpayer as federal and state governments subsidize the meat industry every step of the way. If these costs weren't borne unknowingly by you the taxpayer, but showed up instead at the grocery cash register, the cheapest hamburger meat would be $35 a pound,[92] and that was 14 years ago. If you find that hard to believe, here's what the General Accounting Office, the Rand Corporation and the Water Resources Council had to say:

"...it is clear that irrigation subsidies to livestock producers are economically counterproductive. Every ($1) dollar that state governments dole out to livestock producers in the form of irrigation subsidies, actually costs tax payers seven ($7)....the 17

[90] Ensminger, M.E. "Animal Science," 9th edition, Interstate Publishing, 1991
[91] Borgstrom, Georg, presentation to the annual meeting of the American association for the Advancement of Science, 1981
[92] Robbins, J.

Western states receive limited precipitation, yet their water supplies could support an economy and population twice the size of their present ones. But most of the water goes to produce livestock, either directly or indirectly. Thus, current water use practices threaten to undermine the economies of every state in the region."[93]

If the people living in the Pacific Northwest (Oregon, Washington, and Idaho) had any idea how much it was costing them I wouldn't be surprised if it started a revolution! Not only do livestock producers deplete the state's electrical power capacities, they use enormous power to pump the water to their point of use. All told economists have calculated the three state area loses 17 billion kilowatt hours a year to the gluttonous livestock producers. That's enough to light every house in the entire United States for a month and a half. Does it get any better further south in sunny California known for its abundant fields of strawberries and artichokes; its miles and miles of oranges, lemons, avocado, and grape vineyards; not to mention the vast acreage of lettuce, broccoli and other life enhancing foods? Forget it! Livestock producers are easily California's biggest water consumer, which again costs everyone (meat-eater and non-meat eater alike) out of their own pockets. Here's a good chart to show you the waste I'm talking about.

Cattleman's Beef Association claims it takes only 441 gallons of water[94] for every pound of beef while the Chairman of the Food Science and Human Nutrition Department of the College of Agriculture at Michigan State says it is 2,500 gallons for one pound of beef.[95] The University of California Agricultural Extension, working with livestock farm advisors got a bit more specific saying it took 5,214 gallons per one pound of beef while it also showed how much water was required for other food stuff.

1 pound of lettuce – 23 gallons

---

[93] Fields, David and Hur, Robin "America's Appetite for Meat is Ruining Our Water" Vegetarian Times, Jan. 1985

[94] "Myths About Facts About Beef Production: Water Use National Cattlemen's Beef Association, on their website

[95] Georg Borgstram, "Impacts on Demand for the Quality of Land and Water" presented at 1981 annual meeting of the American Association for the Advancement of Science

1 pound of tomatoes – 23 gallons

1 pound of potatoes – 24 gallons

1 pound of wheat – 25 gallons

1 pound of carrots – 33 gallons

1 pound of apples – 49 gallons

1 pound of chicken – 815 gallons

1 pound of pork – 1,630 gallons

1 pound of beef – 5, 215 gallons[96]

So you might think that all this water consumption at least creates jobs right? Think again – no other industry in the country even comes close to the scarcity of jobs created per gallons of water consumed. For every job created by livestock production in California, it uses 30 million gallons of water a year – far more than the closest competitor.[97]

Economist Douglas McDonald estimates that if water subsidies were withdrawn from California livestock producers, the income of the states other businesses and workers would rise over 10 billion dollars annually. [98] Economists Field and Hur calculate the overall price of California subsidizing the California meat industry to be around 24 billion dollars. That's a thousand dollars for every man, woman, and child in the most populous state in the country – a state that imports most of its meat by the way! Fields and Hur have concluded:

> "whereas the meat industry likes to portray itself as the *backbone* of the American economy, in truth it is more of a *back breaking* burden."[99]

---

[96] "Water Inputs in California Food Production" Water Education Foundation, Sacramento, California
[97] Ibid.
[98] Ibid.
[99] Robbins, J. "Diet.."

What A Waste!

I wish it ended there, but unfortunately the astronomical price keeps growing. Did you know our nations meat habit and the corporate greed of those that would profit from it is creating another huge casualty that most people would never even consider? What do you think happens to all the toxic waste from these animals? Fifty years ago it would have returned to the soil to enrich it and help make compost. No longer, as waste elimination is now a bottom line assembly production meant to get the most bang for the buck. Now it ends up in our water supply! This is no laughing matter as the pile of waste is immense. To give you an idea, in every 24 hour period (the animals soon to be sitting on your table) relieve themselves of 20 billion pounds of waste. There's that word again *waste*. That is seven trillion, three hundred billion pounds a year (7,300,000,000,000 pounds) or a quarter million pounds of manure a second. This is 20 times the amount of the entire U.S. population.[100]

Over half this waste, over a billion *tons* a year, comes from confinement operations from which it can't be recycled. The largest feedlots with 100,000 cattle have a problem equal to that of the most populous American cities. But unlike the residents of New York, L.A. and Chicago, however, they do not pay taxes with which to construct sewage systems. The result – most of it goes into our water supplies. When Newsweek asked the EPA agricultural expert Dr. Harold Bernard about this huge problem, he told it like it is. Feedlot wastes are:

> "….10 to several hundreds of times more concentrated than raw domestic sewage…When the highly concentrated wastes in a runoff flow into a stream or river, the results can be, and frequently are, catastrophic…"[101]

Here's one example:

Gallons of oil spilled by the Exxon Valdez – 12 million

[100] Pimental, David, "Energy and Land Constraints in Food Protein Production" Science Magazine, Nov. 21, 1975 Jasiorowski, H.A. "Intensive Systems of Animal Production" Proceedings from the 3rd World Conference on Animal Production, Sydney University Press, 1975
[101] Newsweek, Nov. 8th, 1971

Gallons of putrefying hog feces and urine spilled into the New
River in North Carolina June 21, 1995 when an 8 acre 'lagoon' of
hog waste burst – 25 million[102]
Fish killed as an immediate result – 10-14 million[103]
Fish whose breeding area was decimated by this disaster – Half
of all mid east coast fish species[104]
Acres of coastal wetlands closed to shell fishing as the result of
this one incident – 364,000[105]
Amount of waste produced by North Carolina's 7 million factory
raised hogs (stored in open cesspools) compared to the amount of
waste produced by the state's 6.5 million people – 4 to 1[106]
Relative concentration of pathogens in hog waste compared to
pathogens in human sewage – 10 to 100 times greater[107]
Consider just the fact that animal wastes account for more than
10 times the amount of water pollution attributed to the entire
human population. Then when you consider that *the meat industry
single handedly accounts for more than three times as much harmful
organic waste pollution as the rest of the nation's industries
combined,*[108] you might think twice before ordering that "double
cheese dead cow patty please." "Oh waitress, while you're at it can
I get a glass of blood also?"
Economists Field and Hur report:
> "A nationwide switch to a diet emphasizing whole grains, fresh
> fruit and vegetables – plus limits on export of non-essential fatty
> foods – would save enough money to cut our imported oil by
> over 60%…a typical household of three could expect to save
> $4,000 a year in the short run. And, if they put aside 30% of
> those savings…the supply of lendable funds from personal

---

[102] Feedstuffs, July 3,1995
[103] Williams, Ted, "assembly Line Swine," Audobon, Mar-April 1998, page 27; see also note 139
[104] Ibid.
[105] Ibid.
[106] Facts and Data, Waste Pollution and the Environment, GRACE Factory Farm Project, www.gracelinks.org
[107] "Environmental and Health Consequences of Animal Factories" Natural Resources Defense Council 1998
[108] Borgstrum, Georg, cited in Lappe, Francis Moore in "Diet For a Small Planet", 1975 edition, page 22

savings would rise 50 percent."[109] Also they add: "Savings on health care alone could be expected to reach $100 billion within 5 years."

I think a good start would be simply if the "Great American Food Machine" in general, and the meat, dairy and egg industries in particular, adopted the policy of the whole truth and nothing but the truth in their advertising campaigns. Then we'd see billboard campaigns so people would know a little more specifically what is happening to their bodies and to their world. How about:

> *"a billion burgers sold, a billion dollar increase in medical costs for cancer and heart attack victims"* or maybe
> *"a billion burgers sold, a billion tons of animal waste enter our water supply"* or maybe
> *"with every billion burgers sold another hundred species become extinct."*

Maybe people just don't fully grasp what extinct means – gone forever, finite, the end, as in never again. Like *Hamell On Trial* reminds us on his brilliant CD *Tough Love*,

> "...what part of 'Thou shall not kill' don't you understand? Thou means you! Shall not means don't!"

Like I said earlier – what a waste, and all for what? So our citizens can become obese and die way before their time, that's what.

If the advertisers won't go that far, how about John Banzhaf's suggestion in a letter to fast-food executives (he's the lawyer who spearheaded the multi billion-dollar lawsuit against the tobacco industry and is now targeting the food machine) that they at least display restaurant signs warning "fatty foods are addictive."

---

[109] Hur, Robin and Fields, David, "How Meat Robs America of its Energy," *Vegetarian Times*, April, 1985

In Conclusion
(The Top 10 Reasons "Jesus' DieT" Is For Everyone)

10. "In regions where...meat is scarce, cardiovascular disease is unknown." Time Magazine

9. Just the grain we feed to fatten up the livestock would feed the entire U.S. population five times over. A full 95% of all our oats and 80% of all our corn goes to feed the livestock.

8. The great forests of the world are being decimated at an alarming rate since grazing is by far the major cause of deforestation. The true cost in oxygen producing trees and our fragile ozone is staggering. That's 1000 animal species a year and one plant species an hour. It seems to me that even one species lost is too much, especially if that one is the cure to AIDS or Alzheimer's Disease. As it is, we'll never know.

7. Ranching and farm factories have become easily the largest drain on our water sources. The water crisis in America could be eased dramatically and probably eliminated altogether with a change in diet. Remember Newsweek magazine: "The water that goes into a 1,000 pound steer would float a destroyer."

6. Our reliance on foreign oil imports would decline just as dramatically as these same water and fossil fuel resources can be put to better use. Let's take it one step further, as expenditures for food and medical care drop in huge amounts from no longer abusing our bodies, personal savings rise along with lendable funds. This lowers interest rates, as does the drop in oil exports which could significantly help pay off our national debt.

5. One of the biggest casualties which few people realize is the depletion of our nutritional topsoil which quite possibly is our greatest natural resource. That alone will take untold decades to recover from, if ever. Years ago I heard that it was a scientific undeniable fact that if we eliminated ants totally from the face of the earth that our planet would become

extinct very quickly, but if we eliminated humans from the face of the earth, the planet would actually thrive. I now understand what they meant.

4. All of this, not to mention the huge lessening of obscene cruelty, horror and torture we inflict on "even these the least of you" as Jesus calls our animal friends. Did you know they have actually done studies on the glandular responses from the terror on cattle and pigs and the rage of the chickens kept in these conditions? I'd be willing to bet that's part of the reason our children have exhibited so much senseless violence the last couple of decades. It only stands to reason when we eat these animals that lived and died so horribly, we consume the toxins triggered by their rage and terror as the poor creatures are being slaughtered.

3. In 1992, sixteen hundred (1600) senior scientists from 71 countries, including over half of all living Nobel Prize winners, signed and released a document titled. **"World Scientists Warning to Humanity."** It begins with the words: "Human beings and the natural world are on a collision course..." They were warning us that we are running out of time and that:

"fundamental changes are urgent if we are to avoid the collision our present course will bring about...a great change in the stewardship for the Earth and life on it is required, if vast human misery is to be avoided and our global home is not to be irretrievably mutilated."

Irretrievably mutilated – think about what that portends! Now you'd think with 1600 leading scientists from around the world releasing a letter like this that it would make headline news in every newspaper in the world. I'm ashamed to say not one leading American or Canadian newspaper even deemed it newsworthy. In all fairness though, the New York Times did find space on the front page for a story about the origins of rock and roll, while Canada's leading newspapers "The Mail" and "The Globe" included a large photograph of cars forming an image of Mickey Mouse.[1] You could say our priorities are a bit askew, or you might even say that's just plain insane!

2. Albert Schweitzer, Gandhi, even Socrates extolled the peace and happiness that comes to people eating a vegetarian diet. In Plato's Republic, when speaking to Glaucon, he says: "and with such a vegetarian diet they may be expected to live in peace and health to a good old age, and bequeath a similar life to their children after them." He goes on to be quite prophetic, predicting both the medical consequences of eating meat as well as the wars that have been fought in its wake between the 'haves' and the 'have-nots.' It's quite the telling prophecy that should be required reading.[2]

...and the number one reason people should become vegetarians.

1. Jesus said so in no uncertain terms, numerous times, in numerous passages reminding us that "Thou shall not kill" was meant for every living thing.

Well folks, what's it gonna be? Now that you know a few more of the facts and can consider the offsetting price that you, your children and your world are paying for these foods, it should be a no-brainer that you'd at least be interested in finding some kind of alternative. Jesus' DieT... is one, but Pritikin, Dean Ornish and others have some great contributions to offer. We all need to make a stand. You're either part of the solution or part of the problem. You're either treating your body as a temple or treating it like a tomb. Now that you know the astronomical quantities of water, energy, grain and land it requires for that burger, is it really worth it? Now that you know a bit about the toxins, hormones and chemicals that end up in your dairy and poultry products, is it worth it? Now that you know almost everything in today's grocery stores is dead food that provides little of the nourishment you and your children require to be healthy, is it worth it? Do you want to continue to eat unnatural foods that are killing you and watch the obesity, cancer and heart disease rates continue to go through the

---

[1] Robbins, John "Diet Revolution"
[2] Plato's "Republic", Book 2, translated by B.Jowett

roof? Do you want to continue to support an industry that violates
basic laws of nature in its cruelty to animals? Do you want your
food to continue to be nuked or do you want to see the food
industry clean up its act and address the problem at its source – the
feedlots?

The choices we make both individually as well as collectively are
going to impact the planet more now than anytime in history.
Nothing less than your personal destiny as well as the destiny of the
planet is up for grabs. What legacy will we leave for our grand-
children? It's up to you to make a choice. We can no longer afford
to sit back and let someone else make the decisions for us. That's
what we've been doing for far too long now and the price has
gotten way out of hand. It's costing us our lives as we collectively
commit a slow suicide.

Don't get me wrong. I've been a meat eater most of my life and
truly understand the allure of a juicy steak, some baby back ribs
smothered in sauce and even the appeal of a good spicy beef jerky. I
have come to realize that though they may be enticing at times, the
price for indulging in them has become more than I'm personally
willing to pay. We each have freedom of choice and I have no
doubt there are many people so addicted to meat, dairy, and egg
products that there is no way in hell they would ever quit entirely,
though, hopefully they will be inspired to cut back considerable.
That's OK too, but you can still demand a healthier product and
start supporting only the companies that use no hormones,
antibiotics and nuclear radiation and that allow their cattle,
chickens, pigs and sheep to graze free range on fields that haven't
been poisoned. Go to any whole foods store and they'll have plenty
of literature on alternatives. Unfortunately the small rancher or
farmer that wants to keep your food healthy doesn't stand much of
a chance against the assembly line factory conglomerates that are
killing us. The reality is, until the public becomes aware of the huge
price we're presently paying to buy that hamburger for 59 cents it's
only going to continue to get worse.

So now that I've hopefully used the motivating factor of fear to
move a few others to action, let's finish solving the rest of the
mystery that inspired this book in the first place.

The Roadmap Ends
Solving The 'Whodunit'

So where did Jesus learn all the wisdom contained within this diet and way of living? How did he know that food heated too high would kill off all its nutrient value? How did he know about the importance of doing enemas? Where did he get the idea to treat women as equals? That was unheard of back then. Did someone teach him? He gave us a moral and ethical system so profound that it is totally relevant today. Where did this profound knowledge that Jesus was able to pass on to mankind originate? Who were his teachers and what was Jesus doing all those years that are unaccounted for?

We all know Jesus was a Jew. Jesus was being taught in the least understood of the three major Jewish sects of that time called the Essenes. There is much available about the other two sects, the Sadducces and the Pharisees, but the Essenes were particularly private as they preferred to be in nature, away from the metropolitan areas. This seems to be another example where there was an enormous attempt to blackout the entire role the Essenes played in the life of Jesus. Some of the early church leaders, in cahoots with the political forces of their day did a fairly thorough job to obliterate this truth. Thanks to Szekely's findings in the Vatican secret vaults, as well as the Dead Sea Scrolls twenty years later, they can now be traced through numerous historical works where their fingerprints are quite obvious. In the only passage where Jesus is mentioned by the highly esteemed and usually very detailed and prolific historian of his time, Flavius Josephus,[1] the forgery is so obvious that even the August Encyclopedia Britannica describes the passage as one:

> "which in its present form has certainly been interpolated or altered, perhaps by a Christian editor, and may indeed be spurious altogether."

Edouard Reuss, one of the greatest and certainly the most sincere and believing of the Christian exegetes, wrote this about that same passage:

---

[1] Flavius Josehus "Antiquities" (Book XVIII, Ch. iii, 3)

"It is with such monstrous interpretations that it is attempted to cover a defeat which only becomes more ridiculous in consequence."

There are numerous authors who wrote about the Essenes, but we have three of the most objective sources from whom we can learn about the first century Essenes. First, Flavious Josephus, the Roman historian born around the same time as Jesus who had an eye for detail as well as an esteemed reputation. Fortunately, Josephus actually became an Essene himself and wrote at great length about their teachings. The second source I found to be quite objective is the Alexandrian philosopher, Philo (also a contemporary of Jesus), who compares the Essenes with the Persian Magi and the great Indian Yogis.[2] And thirdly, Pliny the Elder, who wrote "Natural History" and described the Essenes as:

"A race by themselves, more remarkable than any other in the entire world."[3]

We find it was with good reason that all their contemporary writers regarded the Essenes as a race apart. They were not only different in their principles, but in their daily lives and practices as well. It's almost impossible to find any points on which the numerous authors disagree, in fact, because it's almost unanimous in all accounts it becomes possible to virtually reconstruct not only their lives but their moral concepts as well.

Without exception all the sources agreed that the Essenes had a high moral reputation among not only the various Jewish sects of the time, but among all their neighbors as well. The fact they were held in such high regard is incontestable and there seems to be no unfavorable judgements or opinions recorded against them whatsoever. Szekely discovered in all his research that the Essenes were:

"the only sect to be without enemies and to escape criticism at the hands of even the most censorious writers."

The best source of unedited history about the Essenes would have to come from Flavius Josephus as he recounted his own admission

---

[2] (Quod Omnis Probus Liber, xii-xiii)
[3] Pliny the Elder "Natural History" (V, xvii, 4)

into the Essene Order in his book "Life" some 2000 years ago. Here are some excerpts from his works:

"When I had reached my sixteenth year did I undertake to examine into our different religious sects and their doctrines, that having come to know them I might choose the one that to me appeared the best. I have already mentioned that there were three sects of the Pharisees, Sadducees and the Essenes....Having resolved this, I at once began to prepare myself in different ways that I might be found worthy to be admitted into the Order of Essenes."

"The doctrines of the Essenes tends to teach all men that they confidently may trust their fate in the hands of God, as *nothing happens without His will*. They say the soul is immortal, and they aspire to lead a righteous and honest life."

"They are the most honest people in the world, and always as good as their word. But most of all are those venerated, esteemed and admired who live in the wilderness, on account of the sense of justice that they show and the courage and intrepidity that they manifest in *ever defending truth and innocence*."

"They never keep slaves. They do not think it right that one should be the slave or servant of the other, as *all men are brethren and God the Father*. Therefore, they serve and assist each other."

In Jewish Wars, II, vii, 2-13, Josehus gives us more insights:

"The third class of philosophers among the Jews, and the class that is most esteemed for their just and moral life, is that of the Essenes. They pride highly the strength of mind and the power to *overcome the passions and desires of their natures*."

"They willingly adopt the children of other people and especially while these are very young as they then are most susceptible to teachings and impressions. *They show great kindness to such children,* hold them dear, and teach them all kinds of knowledge and science, morals and religion."

"They do not live in any particular town, but in every town the Order has its respective 'house.' In this 'house' the members take their abode when they arrive on their travels, and they are there supplied with all they want. Everything is there at their disposition, as if in their own houses. There they are received as the best of friends and near relations by persons they never saw before. In every town there is an Elder who has in his care clothes and other necessary things that he *graciously distributes to those who need such.*"

"Before the sun rises and greets the earth with its beams, they do not speak of earthly matters, but read and send forth the sacred, humble prayers that they learned from their fathers. The Elder points out the work in which each one is most skilled. Having thus worked they again gather, bathe themselves in cold water, and *don a white linen garb.* Having washed themselves they proceed to the special halls of the Order where they proceed, perfectly cleansed, to their eating rooms with the utmost reverence as if they entered the holy temple. Everyone having taken his place in Supreme silence and stillness, the bakers of the Brotherhood enter, distributing a bread to each person. The cook sets before each one a plate of vegetables and other eatables."

"This being performed, one of the priests steps forth and holds a prayer. They consider it a grave sin to rest or touch food before praying. The meal is taken with the most solemn silence and stillness. No noise or dispute disturbs the peace of the house. They talk by turns, and in a low tone, which will appear strange to those not used to it. They eat and drink only what is necessary for their wants."

"In general they do not act without the knowledge and consent of their Elders, but it is always left to their own free will to *exercise benevolence and compassion to all in want, of all classes in society; To feed the hungry, clothe the naked, shelter the homeless; To comfort the sick, to visit, assist and to comfort the prisoner; To comfort, aid and protect the widows and fatherless.*"

"They never let themselves be overcome by anger, hatred, vengeance or ill-will. Indeed, they are the champions of faith, truth and honesty as the servants and arbitrators of peace."

"Their 'Yea' and 'Nay' were with them as binding as the most sacred oath."

"Oaths and profanity are with them as much shunned as perjury itself. They consider that a man loses his esteem among his fellow citizens whose word is not sufficient without swearing."

"They study with perseverance and interest ancient writings, *especially such that are intended to indurate and strengthen the body and ennoble and sanctify the spirit.* They have *profound knowledge of the art of healing,* and study it arduously. They examine and are *acquainted with the medicinal herbs and plants,* which they prepare as medicine for man and beasts."

"Before admittance to the brotherhood one has first to pass a whole year of trials outside the same during which he has to prove himself worthy through a strictly moral and virtuous life and temperance. Having passed through these, *he is sprinkled with water, or 'baptized' as a sign of his spiritual purity and liberation from material things."*

"Above all things to love God."

"They say that during the worldly life the spirit is chained to the body like a prisoner in his cell. But when these chains burst, by wear and decay, then the spirit is freed from the bodily prison."

"Their presages (predictions) often came true, and this increased their esteem with the people as holy men and women. Rightly do they deserve to be called an example for the life of other people."

Josephus also left us with the oath that they asked of every candidate after the three years had expired before being admitted to the communal meal.

"He will exercise piety towards the Deity, and justice towards men."

"He will do no harm to anyone, either of his own accord or by the command of others."

"He will always shun the unjust and cleave to the just."

"He will always show a good example to all men."

"He will show himself loyal to his masters since their power comes from God and his angels."

"He will never force his personal opinion or authority on others."

"He will at no time wear special or luxurious garments."

"He will love the truth and avoid all that is false."

"He will keep his hands clean from all material impurities and his soul free from all unclean thoughts."

"He will never have secrets from his brethren, and he will never denounce them even at the cost of his own life."

"Moreover he swears he will transmit the traditions he has received."

"He will preserve the sacred scriptures, books and traditions with the greatest care."

"He will scrupulously keep the names and commands of the angels, which he has learned to know."

Other first century historians such as the Alexandrian philosopher Philo and Pliny the Elder had interesting observations on the Essenes that are worthy of mention.

They all agreed that the Essenes never ate meat and took no other drink than rain water and the juice of fruits. They also all agree that the Essenes *lived chiefly on the fruits of trees and bushes, and on vegetables and the seeds of the fields*. Also I was delighted to find out that most of the authors mention that the Essenes were fond of music and were always happy. They also all mention that the Essenes *attached great importance to their communal meals* that were always at sunset and were partaken of in silence preceded by special prayer.

The first century Essenes in particular were without exception opposed to life in the big cities and they always lived in the country near lakes and rivers.

They always condemned slavery in no uncertain terms and they lived on terms of *perfect equality between men and women*, contrary to the customs and social structure of the period. The Elders who educated the young enjoyed the greatest respect, but this was not a system of hierarchy.

They enjoyed holiday every seventh day in an atmosphere of joy and contentment and they regarded the evening as the beginning of the day.

All the authors agree that they had secret traditions, practices, and teachings, which were transmissible only by initiaton and they always stressed that to understand their teachings it was necessary to live the true life for many years and to change oneself, physically, intellectually and morally. For this reason they had a three year novitiate before finally accepting anyone among them. The results show that this was an excellent system, as no case of expulsion was ever noted in their history.

So we now have a track record of where Jesus became so learned on the subject of not only physical diet, but our mental, emotional and spiritual diet as well. We also have a track record to follow of what happened when Szekely tried this way of life out on a modern world and found it to be just as effective and potent as it was 2000 years ago. And last, but certainly not least, we now have a road map to follow the track record of The Essenes themselves who were around long before Jesus ever came to be the example for mankind.

And Finally

I know this has been a lot to absorb in one sitting but a few final thoughts to consider that have been touched on throughout this book.

1. The original meaning of the Latin word for religion is 'religare' which simply means to connect. Drawing from that definition, religion might be better served as a quest for knowledge and practicing ways of drawing on all the sources of energy and harmony in the universe.

2. The only dogma that will help bring about the 'peace that passeth all understanding' should be that we never have dogmas. By considering ourselves in possession of the only and exclusive truth, we are not only committing intellectual suicide by separating ourselves from an ever-changing ever-evolving universe but retarding our individual and collective evolutions as well. Those who maintain rigid attitudes, no matter how admirable the philosophy, have closed the door to truth.

3. The essence of each religion is ageless and universal. Unfortunately, the typical sterile mind that is so prevalent in humankind in the 21st century seeks out the safety of dogmas, empty rituals and the outward appearance of ceremony. Mankind would be far better served by adhering to the original purity and simplicity of all the great teachings and avoid the commentaries and commentary on the commentaries that have piled up over the centuries.

4. Just as the Essenes believed and Jesus taught his followers, the essence of any religion is the Brotherhood of Man, The Motherhood of Nature and the Fatherhood of God, keeping in mind that "organization is the death of an idea." Instead let us unite *all* the spiritual forces of life together against the forces of death. To do this we need mutual knowledge as that leads to mutual understanding which leads to mutual cooperation which leads to peace.

5. As the Essenes taught also, there are two kinds of pleasures in life – the false temporary pleasures which we end up paying a very high price for in the sacrifice of our physical health and peace of mind without which of course, we are unable to enjoy any pleasures at all. Whereas the true pleasures are enduring, such as friendship and love; the sights sounds and smells of nature; the mountains, the forests, the oceans, the lakes, and the daily magic of sunrise and sunset; and lastly, great books, great works of art, great music. They knew way back then that the wise man's ideal for a creative, evolving life is to gradually replace the false pleasures for the more noble harmonious pleasures of life which are eternal.

6. The only way to improve society as a whole is to improve ourselves and become "practical idealists" as the British historian Toynbee so beautifully put it.

Our aims and principles should be that human beings, regardless of race, color or creed can better themselves. Furthermore, that every individual owes a duty to not only their self, but the community and to the future of the human race as well to make that improvement the most important task of their lives. The surest path to follow is the study of nature as it is God's blueprint prepared for us in all the vibrant colors of the rainbow. This is the path that will lead to beauty over ugliness, truth over error, of good over egotism and the death of hatred. By focusing on the strengthening of the good we can progressively overcome evil.

Life-Generating and Life-Sustaining Foods

Balance among the life-generating and the life-sustaining foods is the goal and is essential to a long healthy life. Remember, you get energy from the good carbohydrates, you rebuild your body with non-taxing proteins while good oils are the lubricant that keep the entire machine running smoothly. Let's start the list with the fruits. They can be eaten fresh or sun dried (dehydrators are great!) and can be used as a meal in itself or as a desert. Always try and find organically grown.

Organic Fruit

Apples	Figs	Papayas
Apricots	Grapefruits	Peaches
Avocados	Grapes	Pears
Bananas	Honeydew	Pineapples
Blackberries	Kiwi	Plums
Blueberries	Kumquats	Prunes
Cantaloupes	Lemons/Limes	Raspberries
Casaba Melon	Mangos	Strawberries
Cherries	Nectarines	Tomatoes
Cranberries	Oranges	Watermelon
Crenshaw Melon		

Note: All dried fruits should be unsulphured. Dry them in the sun during the summer or invest in a dehydrator – you'll never regret it!

Nuts and Seeds

Almonds	Hazel Nuts	Pumpkin Seeds
Brazil Nuts	Hemp Seeds	Sesame Seeds
Cashews	Pecans	Sunflower Seeds
Chestnuts	Pine Nuts	Walnuts
Filberts		

All rich in protein, oils, fiber and micronutrients. Always buy nuts in the shell as they are much fresher. To be eaten raw and unsalted or blended into nut butter, nut milk, etc.

Organic Vegetables

Alfalfa Sprouts	Cucumber	Peppers
Artichokes	Dandelion Greens	Potatoes (sweet)
Asparagus	Eggplant	Radishes
Beets	Endive	Shallots
Bean Sprouts	Escarole	Spinach
Broccoli	Garlic	String Beans
Brussels Sprouts	Green Peas	Squash
Cabbage	Kale	Swiss Chard
Carrots	Leeks	Tomatoes
Cauliflower	Lettuce	Turnips
Celery	Mustard Greens	Wheat Grass
Chives	Okra	Watercress
Collards	Onions	Yams
Corn	Parsnips	

Legumes

Beans (dozens of varieties)	Lentils
Black Beans	Lima Beans
Black Eye Peas	Navy Beans
Chickpeas (humus)	Pinto Beans
Garbanzo beans	Red Kidney Beans
Great Northern Beans	Split Peas
Green Beans	Soybeans

Note: Rich in protein, especially soybeans

Natural Sweeteners

Barley Malt	Pure Maple Syrup (Grade B)
Blackstrap Molasses	Rice Syrup
Date Sugar	Stevia (herb) my favorite
Fruit Juices-concentrate	Unsulphured Molasses
Honey (raw, unprocessed)	

Natural Oils

Almond Oil	Sesame Seed Oil
Flaxseed Oil	Soy Oil
Peanut Oil	Sunflower Oil
Pure Organic Olive Oil (the best)	Walnut Oil
Safflower Oil	

Note: These are all unsaturated and allowable. Stay away from any oils that contain chemical additives. Cold pressed and expeller-pressed are the best and can be found at most health food stores.

Natural Whole Grains, Flours & Cereals

Amaranth	Flax
Barley (whole)	Oats (steel cut oats)
Basmati Rice	Quinoa
Brown Rice (natural unrefined)	Rye
Buckwheat	Whole Wheat (unbleached)
Bulgur	Wild Rice
Corn Meal (yellow, white, blue)	

Note: For cereal use any of the natural sweeteners and soy milk, almond milk or rice dream.

3 Sample Menus

For those on the transition diet still eating three meals daily.

Menu 1

Breakfast

Fresh fruit to start. Hot slow cooked oatmeal or other whole grain cereal or granola, with banana, peaches or berries on top. Sweeten with raw honey or Stevia and use soy milk or rice milk. Herbal tea sweetened with honey or Stevia (optional)

Lunch

Raw veggie salad:

1 stalks celery, chopped	½ cup chopped red cabbage
1/2 bell pepper diced	1 turnip grated
½ cucumber, chopped	½ cup sunflower seeds
1 carrot (grated)	(for variety add mushrooms,
1 beet (grated)	sugar pea)

Dice 1 avocado and 2 tomatoes and use as a dressing. Mix thoroughly and serve on bed of lettuce, spinach or cabbage leaf. Apple cider, olive oil, garlic, raw honey, w/ fresh herbs mixed with lemon or orange is a heavenly dressing

Bowl of vegetable or bean soup. Fresh fruit or homemade fruit leathers or banana dipped in carob for dessert.

Dinner

Another raw vegetable salad. Beans tempeh, soy, tofu or humus for protein. Two cooked vegetables. Fresh fruit, soy yogurt, wholegrain cookie for dessert.

Menu 2

Breakfast

Fruit Smoothie w/ everything prepared in a blender.

Start with fresh squeezed orange juice, grapefruit, tangerine or tangelo, unsweetened pineapple juice or water. For variety use vegetable base of carrots.

Two ripe bananas and/or any seasonal fresh fruit such as pears, peaches, strawberries, apples, apricots, dates etc. (in winter – frozen organic fruits are fine)

Add: ½ tsp. raw wheat germ
½ tsp. lecithin granules
½ tsp. rice bran
½ tsp. wheat germ
½ tsp. soy protein
½ tsp. vitamin C powder
½ tsp. nutritional yeast flakes
1 tbsp. raw sunflower seeds
1 tbsp. raw (not processed) honey
1-2 tsp. barley green powder
1 tbsp. psyllium husk powder (optional)

Lunch

Another variety fresh raw salad, soup or veggie-burger, steamed yellow squash.

Dinner

Raw vegetable salad w/healthy dressing, green, yellow or red bell pepper stuffed with brown rice, and a flavored tofu. For those still transitioning from a dead food to a life food regime get rid of the red meats entirely and eat only fish high in Omega 3 oils such as tuna.

Menu 3

Breakfast

Another smoothie (there are countless combinations so you never get bored); or fresh fruit, fresh range free fertile egg, 2 slices whole grain toast or try blue-corn pancakes and waffles for a variety. Homemade yogurt (preferably soy yogurt) with bananas and honey, or berries, or frozen orange juice (one of my favorites).

Lunch

Raw vegetable salad, corn on the cob or stewed fresh tomatoes, or brown rice casserole which has everything. Fresh fruit and nuts for dessert.

Dinner

Raw vegetable salad. A vegetable protein, sweet or baked potato, yellow squash or bowl of steamed spinach with tomatoes. Dessert – fresh fruit with yogurt, homemade blackberry cobbler or apple pie (substituting stevia for sugar).

Stay tuned for *Jesus' DieT For All The World*
Recipe Book due out in 2006

Twelve Reasons to Experience Gene Wall Cole Through His Books, Music and Workshops

Praise for visionary thinker, life-long adventurer and musician extraordinaire Gene Wall Cole as he has been Awakening Imaginations throughout the world.

"Gene's music is the first meeting between East and West in a musical vibration; it will heal many people."

– The Dalai Lama

"One of the most defining moments of Grace at the HOPE 2000 conference was Gene's personal testimonial and the philosophy of life he shared with us that day. It touched many delegates and made it evident to all that the higher power for all of us worked in many strange and beautiful ways. May you continue to dazzle all and touch many more with your loving spirit and concern."

– United Nations Drug Control Program,
Dr. Anand B. Chaudhuri MD

"Gene has a great talent and I enjoyed his artistry immensely. When he asked me for a quote I thought of Proverbs 3:4-6: "So shalt thou find favor and good understanding in the sight of God and man. In all ways acknowledge him and he shall direct thy path." – Billy Graham Evangelical Association
Rev. Henry Holly

"Gene Wall Cole is the epitome of a vessel of enthusiasm, inspiration and a willingness to be used as an instrument for good on our planet at this time. The music that he sings, the spontaneous humor that flows through him and the joy in his soul is the evidence that the presence of God is real, for him – as him – he's a Reverend for God!

– Rev. Michael Beckwith
founder of Agape International Center for Truth;
President of Association for Global New Thought

"Gene Wall Cole is one of the most motivated individuals I have
ever met. He set a new performance standard at my company. In
less than a year he almost doubled the existing sales record at
Investors Business Daily! His drive and determination are a thing
of legend."

– Investors Business Daily,
William O'Neil, Owner and CEO

"If you're into listening to a guy who is tuned on to a higher level
wisdom, then you'll enjoy the man, his music and reading his
books."   – Mark Victor Hansen,

#1 New York Times author
of *Chicken Soup for the... Series*

"Gene is an old friend and a new brother. He was already on the
path when we first met nearly 20 years ago. You're in for a treat!"

– Marianne Williamson,
#1 New York Times best selling author

"Gene is an extraordinary man. Knowing him as an artist with
astonishing skills, I anticipated enjoying his music, but was
overwhelmed by the level of sheer invention in both the
production of the music and the writing of *The Chameleon*. His
story is compelling reading, filled with imagination and humor.
His life is inspiring and he has a gift for sharing a sense of hope.
Can't wait to see The Chameleon on the silver screen."   – Shadoe
Stevens,

Actor/Radio and TV personality

"I found Gene's rigorous honesty both courageous and disarming
and his humor most refreshing. I give both his book, *The
Chameleon*, and his ministry, 'Awakening Imaginations' a hearty
two thumbs up!"

– John Bradshaw,
#1 New York Times best selling
author and lecturer

"I have known Gene for a long time and I know him to be a man in search of wisdom and truth. He was one of my 'Guardian Angels.' His creative muse will inspire and delight you as it has me."

– Barbara DeAngelis,
#1 New York Times best selling author

"Gene's multi-media book, The Chameleon, was inspired from his 'Artist's Pages' and is the first of its kind. Gene has followed his heart and his art. He is a true original."

– Julie Cameron,
best selling author, *The Artist's Way*

"I know Gene Wall Cole. Please read his book! I was one of the first people he shared it with as he too has experienced coming back from the other side. He knows his part."

– Dannion Brinkley,
#1 New York Times best selling author

A Guide To

THE QUICKEST,
MOST NATURAL
WEIGHT LOSS PROGRAM
AVAILABLE

A Wake-Up Call To

OPTIMUM HEALTH
AND PEACE OF MIND

A Roadmap To

SOLVING THE
GREATEST 'WHODUNIT'
IN HISTORY

To book Gene For Keynotes, Seminars, Concerts and Workshops
Contact The Awakening Imaginations Foundation:

National Program Director
Awakening Imaginations
P.O. Box 344
Henrietta, NC 28076

Telephone 828-657-5416

e-mail awakening1@bellsouth.net
Website www.genewallcole.com

Also By Gene Wall Cole

Books:

You May Be Right, but CONSIDER THIS... –

Musings of a Spiritual Truckdriver Fasting From Ignorance.
His just completed seven year work of love about the
evolution of ethics, democracy, and spirituality, or as Gene
prefers to call it A 40 Day Fast From Ignorance on Life
Liberty and the Pursuit of Happiness.
The Foreword was written By His Holiness The Dalai
Lama

Advance Praise for *Consider This*

I just finished reading *You May Be Right, but Consider
This...* by Gene Wall Cole. My initial reaction – WOW –
easily one of the most thought-provoking books I've ever
read! It also inspired laughter so hard tears were running
down my face!
• intelligent, but not heady
• well researched, but not tedious
• humorous, yet respectful
• very readable
• excellent conversational tone
• well organized into bite sized nuggets, yet tied together
  in a cohesive message on the current condition of our
  country and our world
• great cross disciplinary references and perspectives
• if marketed correctly, definitely a best seller which will
  have greatest impact on the concerned and confused
  masses, who know something is terribly wrong in our
  country and our world, but have no idea what it is or
  what to do about it
After Day 17 I wanted ten copies to give to friends in the
world – after Day 27 I requested copies to give to all the
executives at Cisco – by Day 39 I decided to create an
approach where I could get it in the hands of our CEO

personally, as Cisco's motto is, "changing the way the world works, lives, plays and learns" and *Consider This...* speaks to all four magnificently.

Lisa G. Jing
Human Resources Manager, Worldwide Diversity
Cisco Systems, Inc.

Excerpts from *Consider This*

"Beyond the place of right thinking and wrong thinking
there is a field—I'll meet you
there"   Rainer Maria Rilke

Human truths, like everything else in nature, evolve and have their birth, growth and decline. An elementary school child today probably knows more than the sages of ancient Greece and Rome, while the child of tomorrow will know more than the wisest of us. We once thought the earth was flat, until someone reconsidered that belief. We once believed the sun rotated around the earth, until Galileo considered another possibility and was pronounced a heretic for his troubles. For those not quite up to date, in 1991 the Vatican finally admitted he was right (only 400 some-odd years late, but hey, better late than never.) The fact is everything evolves! "Consider This..." is about the evolution of ethics democracy and spirituality, or, if you prefer, "life, liberty and the pursuit of happiness."

The driving philosophical principle behind "Consider This..." is based on the belief that the entire history of human culture is the antagonism between 2 points of view – a static world view, and a dynamic world view where everything is constantly evolving. With the advancement of quantum physics and the unraveling of the DNA mystery, we have finally established that everything is made of energy – EVERYTHING! "Consider This..." comes from knowing that this apparent abstract fact has very practical consequences.

I see the static world view as extremely dangerous, and recognize that from this concept has sprung the fanatics of every age. They say "we possess the absolute eternal truth, and all others are false." I believe when these tendencies are in power in politics, there are wars and terrorism. When they hold sway in religion there is fanaticism and persecution. When they take the lead in the realm of science, there comes a sterile period in scientific progress. The fact is, the idea of truth has undergone a progressive disturbance and Einstein, Galileo, Darwin, Hawkings and so many others have proven beyond a reasonable doubt the 'relativity' of all things. One reminder I've kept close throughout this work of love, was a quote by British philosopher and writer Herbert Spencer:

"There is a principle which is a bar against all information, which is proof against all arguments and which cannot fail to keep a man in everlasting ignorance – that principle is contempt prior to investigation."

The Chameleon – A Spiritual Adventure Through Wine Women and Song

Gene's powerful rite of passage growing up in America – A first of its kind multi-media musical memoir complete with 3 CD's of Gene's original music and 75 poems at the back of the book. With an asterisk and footnote on the printed page and a remote for your CD player in your hands, you can hear the music that fits the story and corresponds with Gene's journey.

The much anticipated *Jesus' DieT For All The World Recipe Book* – due out in 2006

Videos and DVD

FOLLOW YOUR DREAMS – THE WORKSHOP
Gene's highly acclaimed 3 hour experiential workshop that
has been received all over the world

Music CDs

RAINBOW CD
Contains the music Gene performed at the service and is
primarily songs about God and one's divinity. In it he covers
all colors of music from Jazz to Dixieland to Classical and
Rock. Using 55 of the world's greatest musicians, it is a
family favorite.

AWAKENING IMAGINATIONS CD
An all-instrumental composition that features the one of a
kind instrument (the Dulsitar) that Gene played at the service
and in the workshop/concert. It is used by meditators,
healers, masseurs and people who want to be surrounded by
gentle acoustic sounds.

CHAMELEON CD
A mix of Classical, Rock, Jazz and a variety of musical
styles all featuring original compositions by Gene. Endre
Balogh is featured on the Stradivarius. This is a perennial
best seller.

STAIRWAY TO HEAVEN CD
A 54 minute guided meditation featuring the one of a kind
"Dulsitar," accompanied by world renowned pianist Jeffrey
Lance.

IS THAT THE KIND OF COUNTRY YOU WANT CD
A must have for any country music fan. Featuring Paul
McCartney's drummer, John Lennon's keyboard player and
Merle Haggard's pedal steel guitarist, it is destined to become
a classic.

All of these plus much more available on the website

Conferences, Keynotes, And In-house Seminars

Gene speaks on subjects that he is most passionate about, such as how to gain leadership over your personal and professional life through transformation and realizing your greatest potential. The enormous depth and range of sources that he draws upon have a huge impact because his presentations feature effective strategies that get bottom line results, fast! He always makes a point to emphasize strategies that you and your team can use in the workplace as well as at home.

Gene knows without a doubt, that in this post 9/11 era, filled with a myriad of challenges as well as boundless opportunities, everyone within an organization needs to be a leader to deepen their level of commitment. Gene's presentations are always customized to suit your specific needs and objectives and tailored to fit your organization's mission statement.

PROGRAM TITLE: "Are You Making a Living or Making a Life?: Powerful Practices for Top Performance and Leadership"

In this results-oriented and profound keynote presentation by Gene Wall Cole, participants will learn breakthrough strategies that are used by top performers throughout the world's most successful organizations. He skillfully leads the participants in techniques designed to capitalize on the opportunities that change presents, while creating extraordinary results. Topics include:

* How to know what is important
* How the best managers build a strong workplace
* The importance of selecting for talent
* The importance of defining the right outcome first
* Knowing your strengths and how to "wow" your clients while building long-lasting relationships
* Bottom line: how to apply the steps – a workable guide

PROGRAM TITLE: "How to Gain Leadership Over Your Life"
In this most memorable presentation, Gene Wall Cole shares the most important lessons he has learned about living a life of authenticity. Drawing from his personal experiences, this program is an intimate look at how others can turn lemons into lemonade, while creating a successful life they've only dreamed of before now. Your audience will learn:

* The importance of following your dreams while being true to yourself
* How to recognize and break those patterns that are limiting your vision
* Bottom line techniques to deepen your personal and professional relationships
* The importance of discipline to achieve personal excellence
* How finding true happiness in our society is a serious problem that must be addressed before one can achieve our heart's desires

For Gene's schedule, bookings, keynotes, concerts, adventure trips and /or further information, contact: Awakening Imaginations National Program Director at (828) 657-5416 or send an eMail to "awakening1@bellsouth.net".

About
THE Awakening Imagi-NATION

Awakening Imaginations began the full time work of inspiring
and motivating people to follow their dreams more than 10 years
ago and has recently been approved for non-profit, tax exempt
status. In that time we have visited more than 40 states, numerous
countries, and have directly impacted literally hundreds of
thousands of lives world-wide. With the release of our founders
new books, CONSIDER THIS, and Jesus DieT For All The World,
and the new workshops, concerts and outreach programs he's
developed, we hope to make a difference in millions more.

THE Awakening Imagi-NATION, is a growing community where
we take literally Einstein's admonition that "Imagination is more
important than knowledge." We are changing the way the world
works, plays, learns, creates, and evolves while guiding people to
rediscover their birthright – HAPPINESS. Money they have, it's
peace joy and happiness they seek.

WE are making a difference one person, one organization, one
event at a time. WE inspire not only individuals but corporations to
see the value of an altruistic long range view instead of just looking
at the bottom line. WE are a positive influence on not only those
around us but on society as a whole. WE bring enormous joy to
those looking for hope and encouragement. WE help those in
recovery from drugs and alcohol as well as those with Attention
Deficit Disorder by sharing our experience, strength and hope with
them. WE are reaching out to children of all ages but especially
high school and college students to help them follow their dreams.

Using language, books, video, and websites to impart the message
of who we are and what we have to offer is almost a contradiction
in itself. It is hard to impart a path of becoming conscious with
mere words, as it has to be experienced. True peace of mind,
wisdom from knowing instead of simply believing, contentment,
awe and an awakening consciousness simply have to be experienced
first hand. But when you have found water in a desert full of thirsty
people, you have to shout – THERE IS WATER HERE!

The broad range of "ministering" products, organizations and
churches, the never ending "self-help" books in bookstores that are

growing annually, and the facts and statistics of the public domain, all demonstrate that people are constantly struggling with problems and issues that tear away at the substance of their lives. No matter how "normal" our childhood, how great our parents, how much or how little money we had growing up or how much education we have, people almost always feel like there is something "missing" in their lives. In spite of this feeling, most people do not reach for, or achieve, their highest dreams and potentials. Why don't we? It is because we think it is impossible. We do not believe that there is a way for us to manifest our deepest desires and follow our dreams...nor do we think we are worthy, and because we do not see a way before us... we give up.

After centuries of spoon feeding by elders, society, and religion, most people are insensitive to taste life first hand, and have no idea when or from where they got their opinions, nor really even care as long as they are approved of. Whether it's food or ideas, the goal is to get true nourishment, and much of the world doesn't know the difference between fresh and canned anymore.

Those in THE Awakening Imagi-NATION community demonstrate and teach others the fundamental elements of happiness and harmony and have the ability to arouse passion for truth, which is a requirement for deeper inner discovery. We are learning to speak with an uncanny logic that can't be denied, but with an inner knowingness and ecstasy that portrays deeper meaning.

WHAT?   We are serving the world by empowering people to become fully alive.

WHY?   Because it brings us happiness and because the greatest thing you can offer the world is being a joyous person.

HOW?   Since people are social creatures and don't want to do it alone, we offer one day, three days, and week long seminars, keynotes for corporations and health organizations, cruises, concerts and coaching. Our on-line worldwide community's sole purpose, is to uncover, discover, and discard old worn out patterns and belief systems that no longer serve us and to be happy anyway.

This will be done using the universal languages of music and humor to open hearts and then by planting seeds of wisdom to help in the prevention of truth decay.

About Gene Wall Cole

Gene Wall Cole is a most amazing and eclectic fellow. Gene is known as a visionary thinker, an author, a speaker and a motivator; a composer, scholar, performer and musician extraordinaire; a metaphysician, storyteller and life adventurer who has always followed the beat of his own drum. Gene Wall Cole is all this and more. In short, he is a true 21st Century Renaissance man. Like the title of his first book, *The Chameleon,* he has the ability to blend in anywhere and has been described as an alchemist of sound, an architect designing a more user friendly world, a sculptor helping people mold their dreams into reality, and a painter whose easel holds the colors of an awakened imagination.

Gene Wall Cole is fast becoming known as one of the nation's leading 'Truth' advocates, better known as a 'consumer advocate.' Described as an Average Joe, who happens to have an insatiable curiosity for knowledge, there's little that doesn't pique his curiosity. An average Joe who has always rooted for the little guy – the underdog – and believed in the idea of fair play. A 'let's have a fair fight and may the best man win' kind of Joe! The kind of Joe who gets bugged because our national pastime has evolved into something the New York Yankees can buy most of the time and wants to know what can be done to fix it. His search for knowledge is voracious, but especially things others might want to keep hidden from an Average Joe. That's his real passion.

Aptly described as Robin Williams/Will Rogers meets Victor Borge/Charles Kuralt, with a touch of Deepak Chopra thrown in for good measure, Gene is a visionary, an author, a speaker, composer, teacher, metaphysician, motivator, and musician. An architect designing a more user friendly world; a sculptor helping people mold their dreams into reality; a painter whose easel holds the colors of an awakened imagination and uses the spoken word as his paint brush. In short, a 21st Century Renaissance Man.

On his innovative website, www.genewallcole.com, his mission statement says it all: "Using the universal languages of music and humor to open hearts, and then planting seeds of wisdom to help in the Prevention of Truth Decay."

Today Gene is everywhere; in concert halls, corporations, churches of all faiths, and meeting halls filled with at-risk kids; at international conferences, on radio and TV, in the recording studio, and behind his computer hammering out new books to shine a bit of the truth he has uncovered and discovered during his amazing sojourn. Much of his time is spent on the road traveling into the hearts of thousands of people each year.

He currently lives in North Carolina with his dog Snudge 'Bullwinkle' Ripley, and was quoted saying "I really need to get a real life" but until then…he's wandering the blue highways of the world uncovering, discovering and discarding worn out beliefs that no longer serve the world.